… The Best of Joe Weider's

MUSCLE & FITNESS
Bodybuilding and Conditioning for Women

The Best of Joe Weider's
MUSCLE & FITNESS
Bodybuilding and Conditioning for Women

Contemporary Books, Inc.
Chicago

Library of Congress Cataloging in Publication Data

Main entry under title:

Bodybuilding and conditioning for women.

   (The Best of Joe Weider's *Muscle & Fitness*)
   1. Bodybuilding for women—Addresses, essays,
lectures.   I. Weider, Joe.   II. *Muscle & Fitness*.
III. Series.
GV546.6.W64C66   1983   646.7′5   83-10138

All photos courtesy of the IFBB.

Copyright © 1983 by Joe Weider
All rights reserved
Published by Contemporary Books, Inc.
180 North Michigan Avenue, Chicago, Illinois 60601
Manufactured in the United States of America
Library of Congress Catalog Card Number: 83-10138
International Standard Book Number: 0-8092-5501-4

Published simultaneously in Canada by Beaverbooks, Ltd.
195 Allstate Parkway, Valleywood Business Park
Markham, Ontario L3R 4T8 Canada

Contents

1   The Heroic Ideal: It's Our Turn
    by Claudia Cornwell Wilbourn

5   Love Thyself
    by Betty Weider

11 My Thoughts on Figure Shaping
    by Claudia Cornwell Wilbourn

13 Workouts Energize Every Cell in Your Body
    by John Howell

15 How Well Do Women Adapt to Exercise?
    by Armand Tanny

17 Getting the Most from Your Health Club
    by Kristine Randal and Joy Grau

20 Body Sculpture and Muscularity: Two Separate Events for Women?
    by Joe Weider (Pro) and Sheila Herman (Con)

25 The Will to Win!
    by Laura Combes

29 Winning Takes More Than Muscle
    by Sheila Herman

33 Surviving a Contest Diet
    by Claudia Cornwell Wilbourn

37 Diuretics: Looking Ripped Could Do You In!
    by Dr. Lynne Pirie, D.O.

41 Female Factors in Bodybuilding
    by Dr. Lynne Pirie, D.O.

45 "We're Training Partners and Proud of It!"
    by Claudia Cornwell Wilbourn

51 A Strong, Sensuous Back
    by Lisa Elliott

59 Conkwright on Posing
    by Betty Weider

63 Rachel McLish: "Variety Is My Spice of Life"
    by Bill Reynolds

69 Energy: Keep Yours at Muscle-Building Levels
    by Raymond Schuessler

77 You Can Create a World-Class Waist
    by Candy Csencsits, as told to Bill Reynolds

83 Shaping the Chest—Kike Elomaa Style
by Rick Wayne

87 "Look at These Shoulders"
by Dr. Lynne Pirie, D.O.

91 "My Armful of Secrets": Mary Roberts' Arm Training Routine
by Sheila Herman

95 Energize Your Legs!
by Rachel McLish

99 These Legs Stop Traffic
by Bill Dobbins

The Best of Joe Weider's
Muscle & Fitness
Bodybuilding and Conditioning for Women

The Heroic Ideal:
It's Our Turn

by Claudia Cornwell Wilbourn

"Woman is subject to man because of the weakness of her mind as well as of her body," claimed a medieval scholar. But what about the heroines and goddesses of literature and legend, from Cleopatra to Isis and Athena? We all know how false the scholar's comment is, yet the myth of feminine frailty and inferiority has prevailed, and the heroic female image is minimized to this day.

If defying cultural limitations, if striving to fulfill genetic potential and refusing to compromise is not heroic, just what is? No group of modern women is more qualified to join the ranks of heroic females than bodybuilders.

Yet the mass media, although fascinated with female bodybuilders as strong, dedicated women, have been reluctant to portray us as descendants of great women achievers. Instead of drawing attention to our strength, sensuality, pride and assertiveness, the media have concentrated on the extremes of our physical endeavor.

In the early days of the sport, for example, Lisa Lyon, Stacey Bentley and I found ourselves constantly before microphones and cameras. We were a curiosity to the journalists, and at one point *People* magazine sent out a crew to Santa Monica to photograph us. They took shots of us basking in the sun, running, weight training, and also wearing evening gowns. When the photos were published, we were shocked to see images emphasizing the extreme details of our regimen—fierce grimaces made during weight training, close-ups of striations and vascularity.

I for one feel betrayed by journalists who miss the very essence of the woman bodybuilder. She is not a freak or a glamour queen or a man-hater. She is a woman in the fullest sense—sensual, proud and strong, defying tradition and daring to reach for physical perfection. This is how she deserves to be portrayed.

I distinctly remember participating in ABC's TV movie *Hustler of Muscle Beach*, featuring Tim Kimber of Gold's Gym. Several male and female bodybuilders were cast in the film, including Lisa Lyon, Stacey Bentley, Frank Zane and Steve Davis. Stacey and I had fun playing ourselves and performing a duplicate posing routine as well as joining the cast in publicity photos. When a publicity photo for the film appeared in *TV Guide*, the images of Lisa, Stacey and myself had been carefully excised and replaced with likenesses of soft, round-hipped models! All other cast members, including the male bodybuilders, had remained in the photo, yet someone upstairs had decided that female bodybuilders were not acceptable or appealing to the American public!

Male bodybuilders easily fit the public's image of heroic figure. They epitomize the cultural

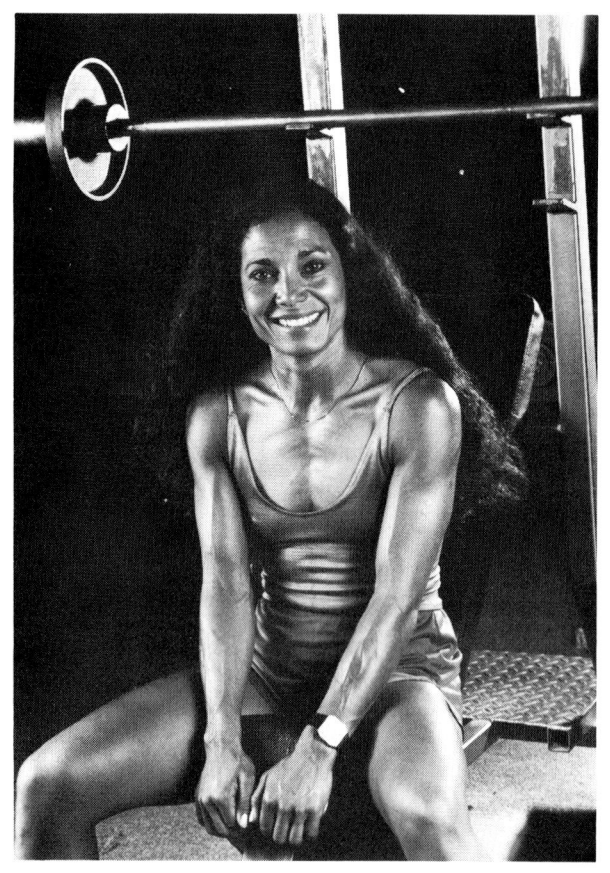

Maria Gonzalez.

ideal of what a man is expected to be. The worship of ferocious male power, superhuman strength and aggressive virility has never waned—from Homer to Hemingway. In more recent times, when the heroic figure is depicted in films and illustrations, a male bodybuilder is usually chosen as model. The heroic film genre blossomed with Steve Reeves, a bodybuilder of exquisite symmetry and grace, as he defended helpless damsels against evil rulers and fierce monsters. Most recently, we have seen the great Arnold Schwarzenegger display his sinew and muscle in the film *Conan the Barbarian*.

Heroic tales have always been popular and will remain so, for people need to believe that human effort, vision and hope can overcome all adversity. Our legends and literature reflect this. The popularity of art, films and TV shows depicting male bodybuilders confirms man's age-old need for courage and endurance to combat evil and fight for justice.

Though female bodybuilders haven't been cast as film heroines, let's not forget that the heroic ideal doesn't refer exclusively to men. "How many glorious deeds of womankind lie unknown to fame!" wrote Seneca. For although heroic deeds weren't performed only by men, the men who wrote history and most of literature failed to give women the credit due them. Little girls are not taught of their legacy—of the great warrior queens, artists, pioneers. We have long been deprived of role models and the knowledge of our possible capabilities.

In a traditional patriarchal culture, softness and weakness are attractive in women, who are viewed as inferior helpmates for males. But the people of ancient Egypt, Rome, Greece and other lands expected more of women. For example, the early Celts and Italians admired feminine audacity. A woman was expected to be a partner with her husband in the pursuit of honor and glory. Her courage, pride, independence and nobility were not considered to be unnatural or unfeminine, but complementary to her mate's attributes.

The great Celtic queen, Boadicea of Britain, was highly revered. In 60 AD she was described with admiration:

"She was tall of person, and of a comely appearance; apparelled in a loose gown of changeable colors, the tresses of her yellow

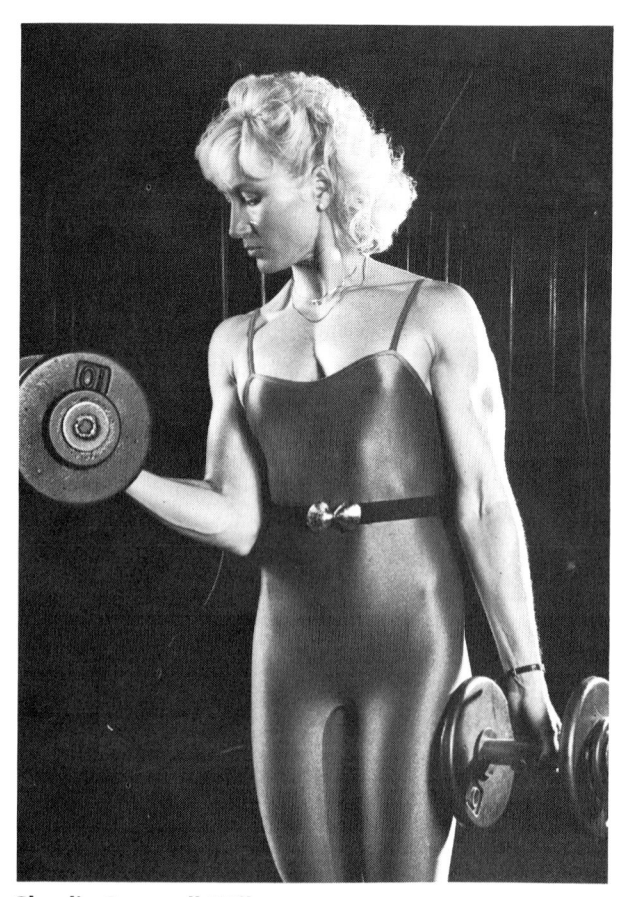

Claudia Cornwell Wilbourn.

hair hung to the skirts of her dress. About her neck she wore a chain of gold, and in her hand she bore a spear. And so for a while she stood surveying her army, and being regarded with a reverential silence she addressed to them an eloquent and impassioned speech."

In the light of such a predecessor, who is better to bind us to the past, to history and a long line of achievers than the female bodybuilder? For the bodybuilder is a pioneer re-creating female heroic endeavors of the past. To a greater extent than males, she dares to go beyond what's expected of her. The very sport of woman's bodybuilding reflects changes in the culture, as do other sports, the arts, politics and business. Female strength, independence and creative pride seen in women bodybuilders are reemerging as desirable qualities.

Women bodybuilders arouse in others an unconscious nostalgia for the heroic feminine ideal. They are strong and sensual, powerful and life-affirming. With an image "bigger than life," they integrate the animal, physical self with the strong, dedicated mind of the athlete.

Fans can be inspired to see women transcending human limitations of age, injuries, genetic inheritance. The female athlete restores lost dignity and pride in womanhood by refusing to accept femaleness as a handicap. The woman bodybuilder is a living metaphor for feminine strength and power and pride.

But a word of caution! While self-knowledge and accomplishment lie at one end of a spectrum, narcissism lurks at the other. Ancient tales recount stories of gods and goddesses destroyed through hubris—wanton arrogance or insolence resulting from excessive pride. The desire for perfection can become obsessive. A woman can attempt to become myth at the expense of her humanity, believing in her exaggerated self-importance. She can deceive herself by creating a fantasy identity. The result can be self-delusion and self-contempt, for a heroic image does not imply superhuman status.

Humility must be cultivated by women bodybuilders. They must realize they owe a debt to good genetic inheritance, to the support and encouragement of others and to the opportunities made available. Today's accomplishments are possible only because of the anonymous women lost to history whose heroic deeds went unsung. Without such predecessors, we wouldn't be here with the strength and determination to succeed.

Heroism doesn't simply mean the slaying of

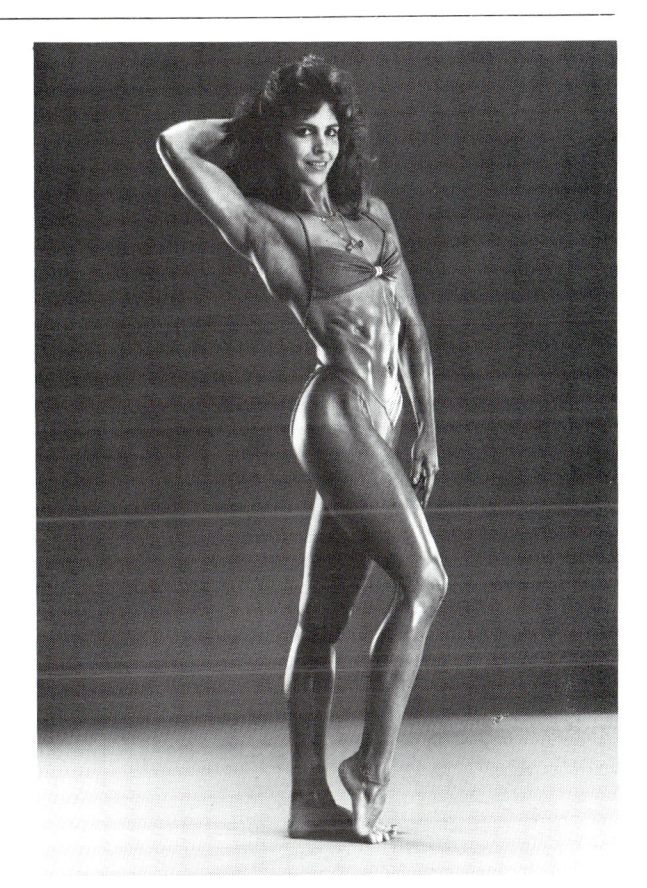

Candy Csencsits.

enemies and the use of violent aggression. Heroism can be doing the most one possibly can. It can be the adding of a significant fragment of accomplishment to the whole of human achievement, making a statement with one's life. It can be resisting the pressure to conform to the feminine stereotype and compromise personal ideals. For the 20th-century heroine does not conquer barbarians and demons, but cultural limitations. She brings meaning to her life by struggling against those who would have women believe in their own frailty.

There does not exist a separate heroism for each sex, but there do exist various facets to heroism. For a woman to adopt a masculine style is to compromise the attributes of womankind. We women can have dreams and goals different from those of men. Woman's morality and heroism is comprised of a responsibility to herself and others and a concern with mercy— "the great adult strength." With this belief that we are all responsible for each other, women contribute empathetic, intelligent caring to the heroic ideal.

Each generation redefines femininity and sets

new standards dating back to prepatriarchal times, when a woman's femaleness was not threatened by her physical strength or intellectual prowess. Frailty and passivity were then viewed as liabilities, as women developed themselves physically, mentally and spiritually.

Today women's bodybuilding is creating its own pantheon of pioneers and achievers. I immediately think of Stacey Bentley and her victory over adolescent fat, Georgia Miller Fudge and her determination to take the role of mother and wife one step further. I think of feline Lisa Lyon with her undiminishing vision of liberation from the feminine stereotype. And I think of Laura Combes, Lisa Elliott and Pillow—women of great muscular density who risk condemnation for their extreme development and personal integrity. I think of all the women in the sport who have overcome surgery, injuries, financial hardships, parental disapproval and structural flaws to dedicate themselves to a vision of physical perfection and athletic prowess. I think of them all as fulfilling the heroic ideal.

Yet female bodybuilders may always be in the vanguard. It takes a special kind of woman to break out of the pack and risk being different. The physical differences between men and women have been exaggerated for centuries through dress, behavior and segregated activities. A female bodybuilder dares to develop her body to the optimum degree and expose its androgynous qualities regardless of the public's acceptance.

I am convinced that women bodybuilders can fulfill the heroic image. With performances of grace and power, they can move audiences, making them think and question their assumptions about male and female—human—limitations. The heroine of the Eighties is not a mythical creature, but a living, breathing woman striving to be the most she possibly can. Today's heroine is more than an exploited body or Hollywood-bound starlet: She is a woman who has dared to live by her own standards of excellence.□

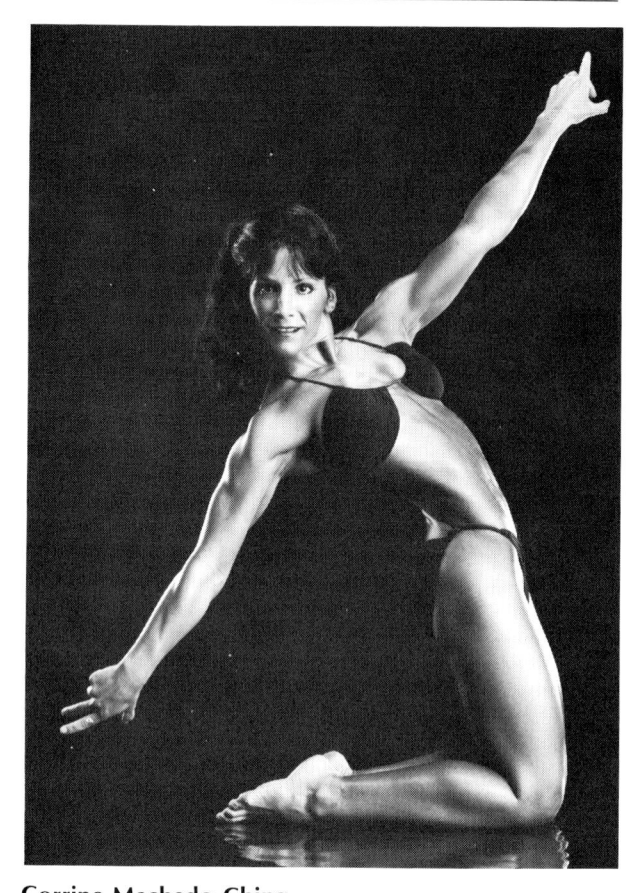

Corrine Machado-Ching.

Love Thyself

by Betty Weider

Watching the World Women's Bodybuilding Championship at Caesars Palace in Las Vegas recently, a friend who was new to the sport turned to me and said, "You wouldn't want to look like that, would you?"

I've heard that question many times and it has always seemed to me that what people really meant was, "Don't you agree that women who display that kind of muscularity look awful?"

Taking that question at face value, I can truthfully say, "I would not want to look like that." The bodybuilding physique, whether for men or women, is very specialized. You can admire it without wanting to emulate it, just as you can be a big fan of gymnastics without wanting to train as a gymnast.

But the underlying criticism implied by the question is more difficult to deal with. A few years ago, when I began to attend women's physique contests, it took me a while to get used to what I saw. Women's bodybuilding is a very recently created sport, and it takes time to learn to appreciate the aesthetics involved. I had always associated muscles with masculinity, so a lot of the women seemed masculine to me. I was not used to women with such low bodyfat, so this lean, muscular look seemed strange to me.

But now I have seen many women's competitions and that feeling of strangeness has worn off. When I look at the women in a contest these days, I can see detail I would not have appreciated before and have a much better feel for the real beauty that a woman bodybuilder's physique can develop.

Nonetheless, I continue to see physiques I don't particularly like. Some women still seem out of proportion to me. But that is, after all, what a physique competition is all about—comparing a number of bodybuilders and judging who's best. Now that I'm more familiar with the sport, I am better able to understand what I'm seeing and can, therefore, exercise my personal taste more appropriately.

However, there are individuals who will continue to dislike the appearance of women bodybuilders no matter how familiar they get with the sport, just as there are people who have never cared much for men's bodybuilding. Everyone has a right to exercise his or her own individual taste.

Taking all this into account, I just smiled when my friend asked her question and waited until after the show, when we were at dinner with my husband, to discuss women's bodybuilding with her more extensively. Actually, it turned out she had enjoyed the competition. She found Rachel McLish, Candy Csencsits and many of the other competitors very appealing, but was disturbed by the more obvious muscular development of some of the others.

6 BODYBUILDING AND CONDITIONING FOR WOMEN

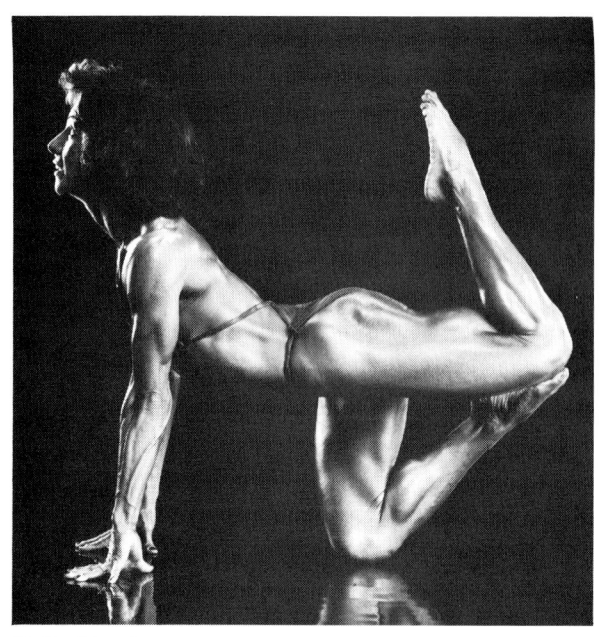

Stella Martinez.

"What you're not taking into account," interjected my husband, "is the difference in women's bodytypes. No matter how hard they try, women who are of different physical types are never going to look the same."

I realized that Joe had put his finger on an aspect of women's bodybuilding that's often overlooked. Our society accepts a wide diversity of male physiques. A pro football lineman like Joe Klecko is going to have a very different kind of build from that of a tennis champion like Jimmy Connors. A rugged-looking man like Sean Connery can make his female audience swoon, but so can a slight individual like Al Pacino.

But we are much less willing to allow diversity when it comes to women's physiques. Society tends to define only a few "acceptable types" in any era, and any woman who is unable to fit the acceptable stereotypes is out of luck.

Going back in history, we can see that this situation has existed for a long time. During the era of the painter Rubens (d. 1640) the acceptable type had a lot of bodyfat. In the 1890's, women were expected to have hourglass figures—big bosoms and hips, tiny waists. The 1920s gave us the flapper—boyish looking, flat-chested, no hips. Later, in the '50s, we admired the lush figure of Marilyn Monroe.

It should be obvious how much fashion in women's bodies changes. But it should also be obvious that women themselves do not change their genetic body types from decade to decade. Women can use diet and clothing to alter their appearance to some degree—if you don't have a natural hourglass figure, for example, you can opt for a whalebone corset, if you can find one—but the fact remains that society selects different types at different times and a look that would make you a celebrated beauty in one era may leave you a wallflower in another.

But why do we accept diversity in men, yet demand that women conform to a limited stereotype? The simple answer seems to be that we understand that men have to look different to accomplish different things—as in the example of the football player and the tennis champion—but a woman's looks are judged by only one criterion: how attractive she is to men.

Now, I am all for women being attractive to men. During the years I worked as a model, it was my business to be as attractive as possible.

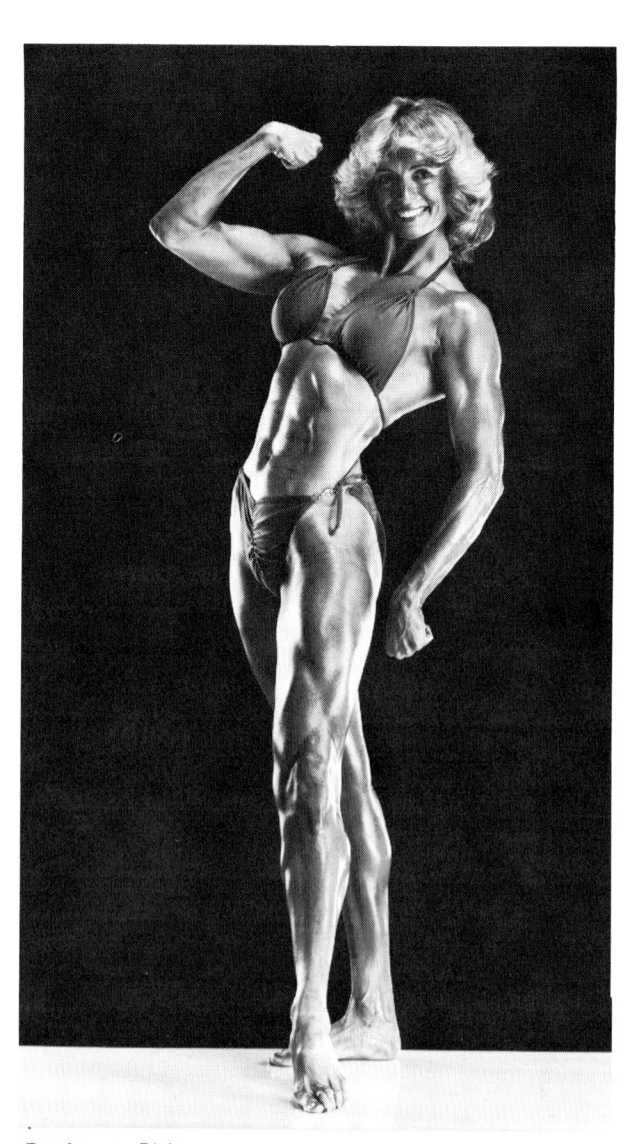

Dr. Lynne Pirie.

Also, I really enjoy the fact that my husband likes the way I look. And I'd like to keep it that way.

We also have to realize that different men have different tastes. Some prefer blondes, others brunettes; some tall women, others short women. The "cultural stereotypes" are matters of public fashion rather than individual preference.

In any sport, what we are looking for is maximum *achievement*—who can run the fastest, jump the highest, perform the feat closest to perfection. In bodybuilding, we look for muscular development that conforms to the highest aesthetic standards of proportion, shape, symmetry, definition and so on.

Assuming that Lillie Langtry, Clara Bow, Betty Grable and Marilyn Monroe all learned to train and diet like bodybuilders, they would certainly

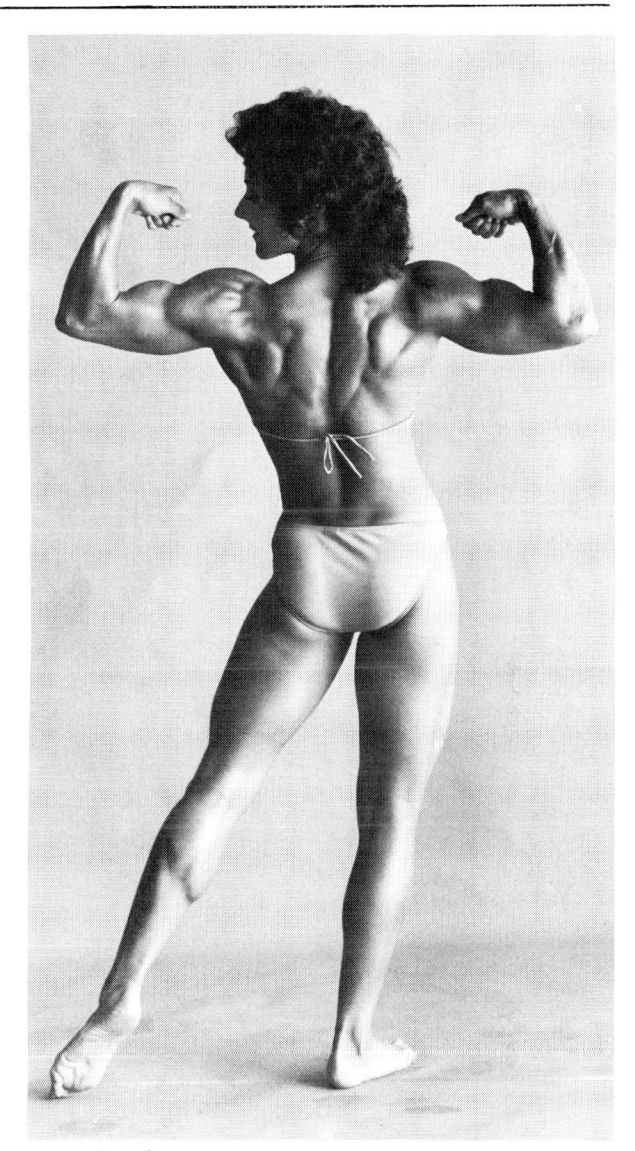

Laura Combes.

not end up looking totally alike —*but they would all begin to look like bodybuilders.* The bodybuilding look is the result of bodybuilding training. The response of the body to this kind of regimen is built in.

You can't really alter the way your body responds to training. All you can do is try to maximize it. Lynn Conkwright can add muscle to her frame, but she'll never develop the muscularity of Laura Combes. Laura can work on improving her symmetry and proportion, but she can't change her basic body type or the structure of her skeleton. So the most each of these women can do is to work on getting the best results she can within the limitations of her genetic heritage.

To be more specific about body types, there is a common system of cataloging the different

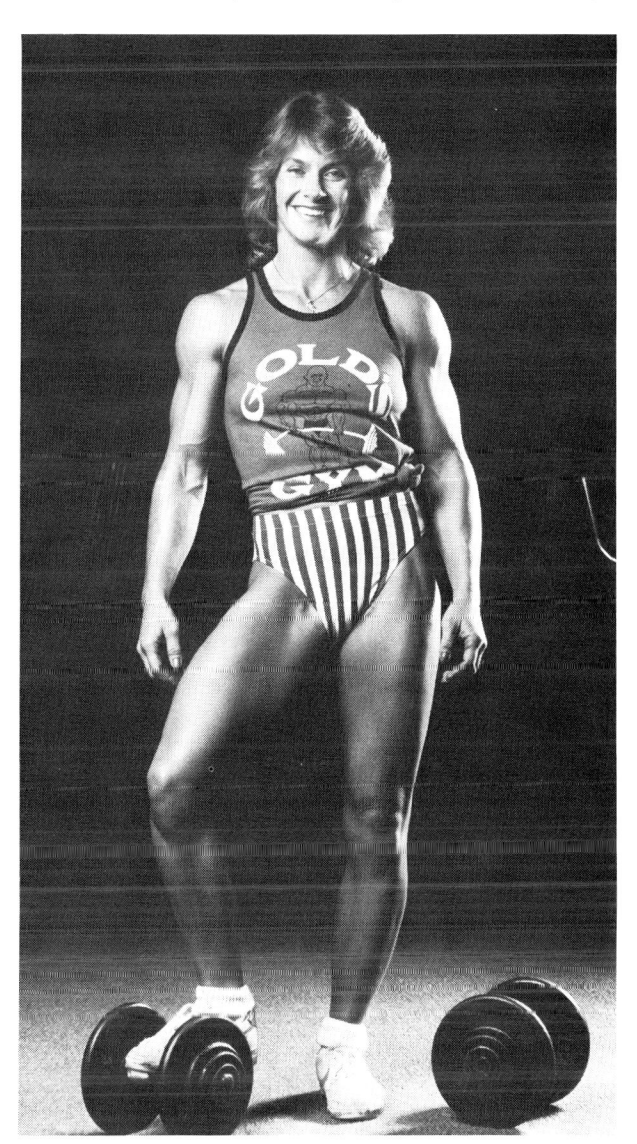

Lisa Elliott.

8 BODYBUILDING AND CONDITIONING FOR WOMEN

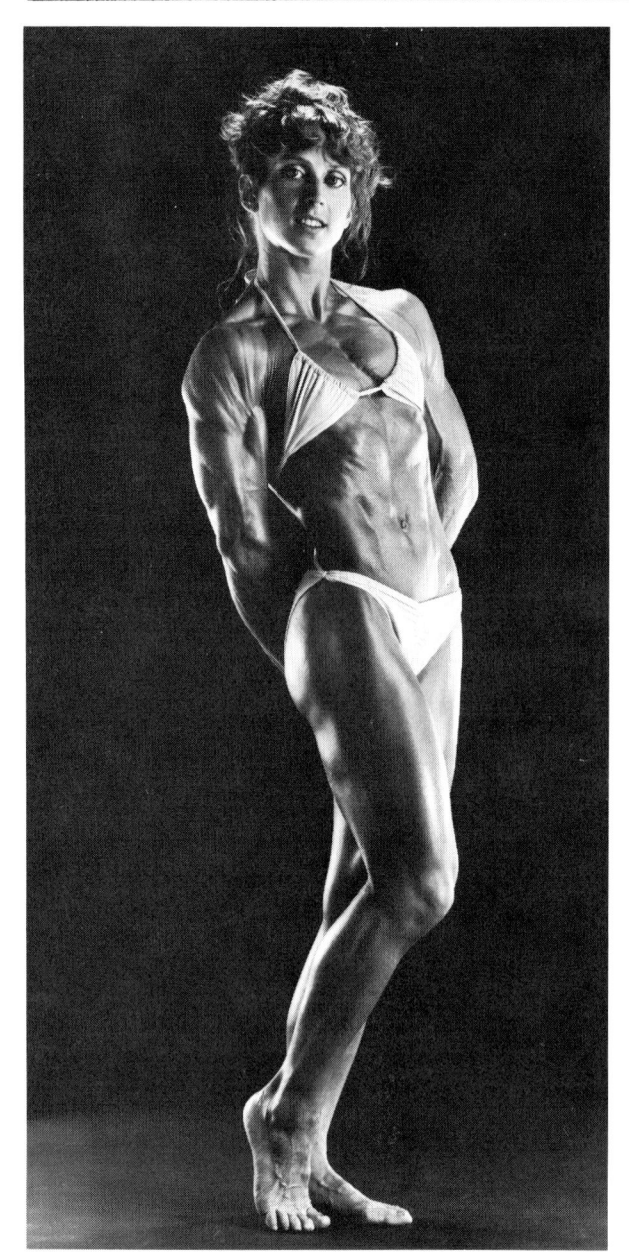

Pillow.

kinds of physiques that uses three basic categories:

- *ectomorph*—long bones, thin musculature, low bodyfat.
- *mesomorph*—heavier skeleton, thick musculature, the "jock" type.
- *endomorph*—soft, round, tending to gain fat easily.

Actually, an individual who is totally one category or another would be very rare. Instead, physiques are rated on a scale of 1-7 according to the degree they possess the characteristics of each of the categories. So a highly ectomorphic *Vogue* model would probably earn:

ectomorphic—7
mesomorphic—3
endomorphic—2

while a Rubens model would more likely be rated:

ectomorphic—1
mesomorphic—4
endomorphic—7

Since this system applies to both men and women, when you see a lineup of women bodybuilders, you can expect quite a variety of combinations of body-type categories. True, to be a bodybuilder means you must be able to build muscle, so most strength athletes will have relatively high mesomorphic quotients.

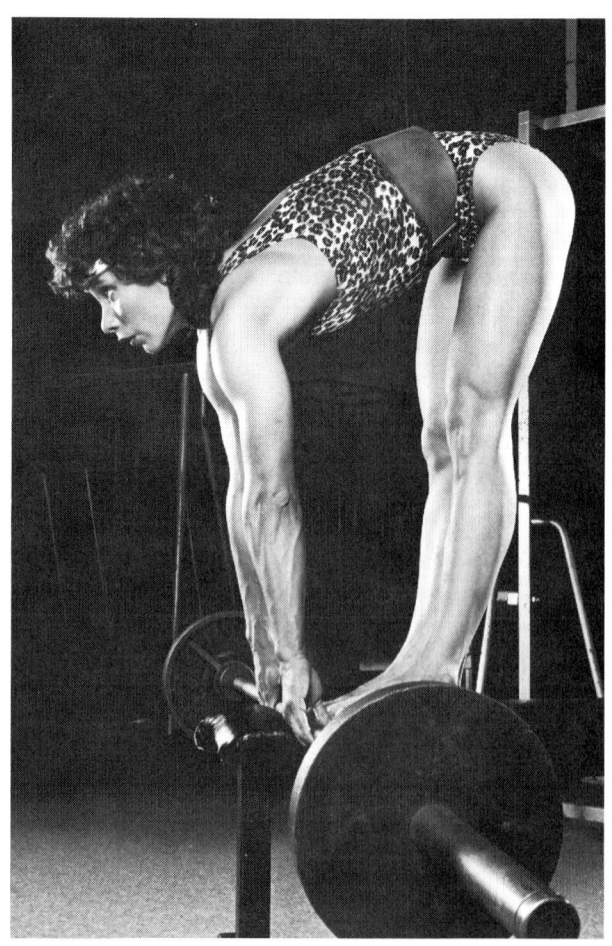

Deborah Diana.

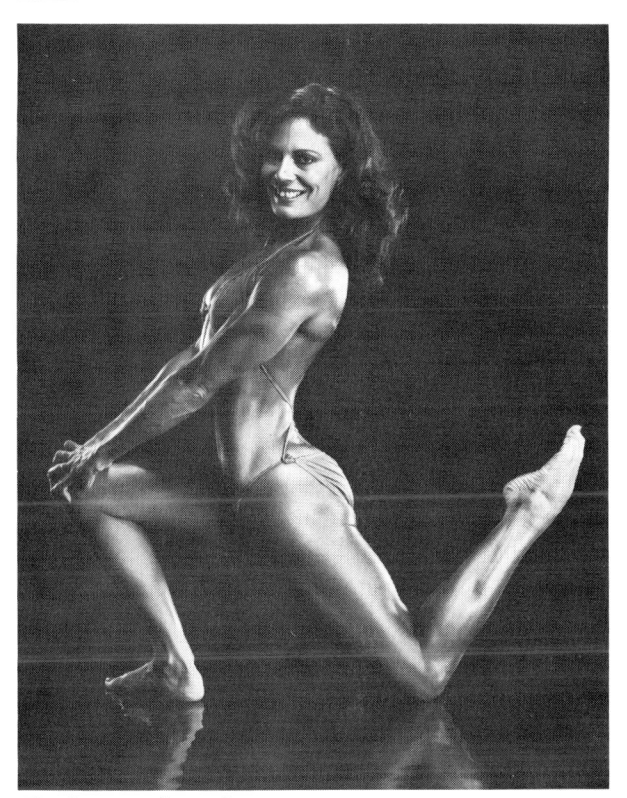

Charlotte Yarbrough.

Nonetheless, you will still see matchups like Claudia Wilbourn and Laura Combes or Lynn Conkwright and Lisa Elliott—obviously all bodybuilders, but very different types.

Of course, the same thing occurs in men's bodybuilding competition. Frank Zane and Mike Mentzer are quite different body types. And since Zane has beaten both Mentzer and Arnold Schwarzenegger, it's obvious that pure muscle size is not the only determining factor in creating a bodybuilding physique.

But there are still more factors to be considered. For example, individuals differ greatly in their natural skeletal proportions. Bodybuilders may have wide or narrow shoulders, shorter or longer arms and legs, different sized hips. People are always complimenting me on my waist. But even though I have always worked very hard with diet and exercise to keep it small, this is a natural genetic characteristic.

Training can be used to some extent to compensate for imperfect genetics. A woman bodybuilder with narrow shoulders can build up her deltoids to correct her proportions. A competitor with a naturally thick waist can avoid building any more abdominal muscle and widen her lats to make the waist look smaller.

Presentation also plays a part in coping with genetics. A woman bodybuilder with short legs can do poses in which a leg is extended to the front, using perspective to make it look longer. A thick-waisted bodybuilder can do a lot of twisting poses, which will make this area look narrower.

All of this is part of the challenge of bodybuilding. There is no such thing as a perfect physique.

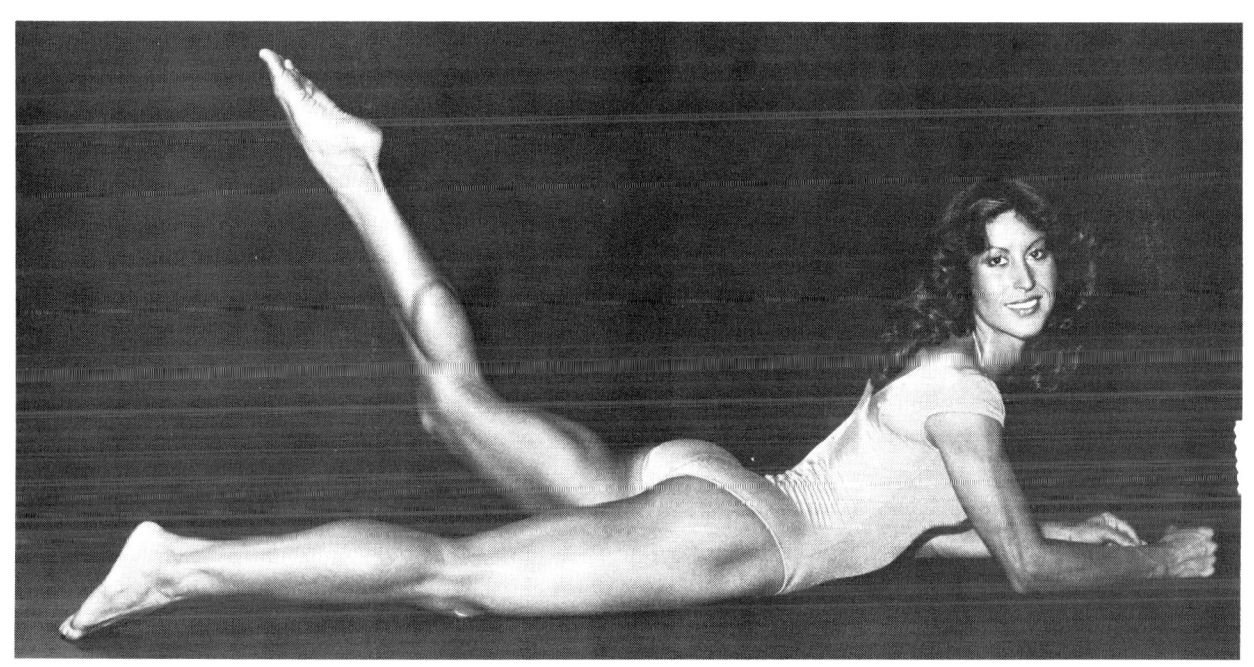

Rachel McLish.

And what this means is that bodybuilding for women allows an acceptance of very different kinds of physiques that far outstrip those of the culture in general. Judging in bodybuilding *does* tend to run in cycles, with one type of physique more in vogue than another. But this is a far cry from the more rigid stereotypes that are imposed outside of bodybuilding on the way women are expected to look.

What we are seeing in the development of first-rate women bodybuilders is a whole range of potential in the female body that we had never realized was there. And this realization has had an effect beyond the competitive level, since gyms are now full of women who may be models, actresses, teachers, housewives and so on, but who are all trying to use these same bodybuilding techniques to achieve their own personal goals.

A woman who does not want to be a bodybuilder is free to opt for a more conventional look. But, on the other hand, a Kike Elomaa, Pillow, Rachel McLish or Kay Baxter is also free to train for competition without being judged inappropriately by standards alien to bodybuilding tradition.□

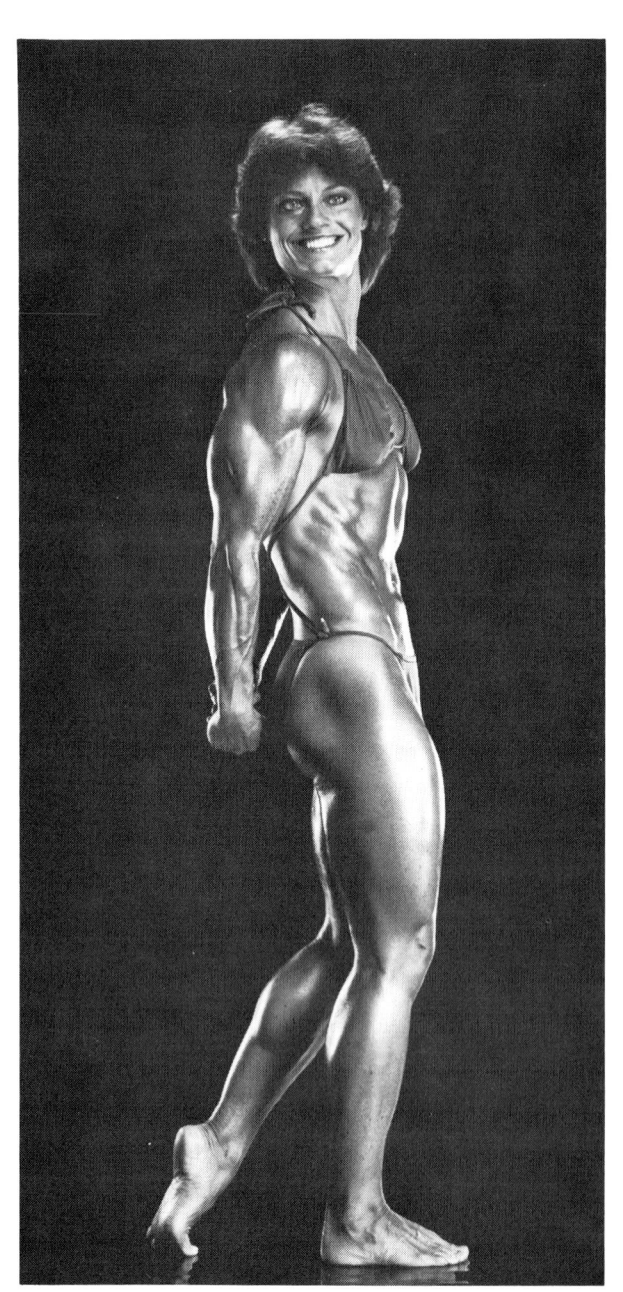

Julie McNew.

My Thoughts on Figure Shaping

by Claudia Cornwell Wilbourn

We women have special bodybuilding problems. We can weight train like men, but we have certain stubborn areas that don't develop the shape and separation we want. Our legs and hips, which can retain three times as much subcutaneous fat as other areas, are the usual trouble spots. Specific weight training exercises are not the answer; diet and aerobic exercise are.

Weight training principles are the same for men as for women. Moderate to heavy weight is needed for deep stimulation. Increased resistance is also needed over a period of time for further development. Squats, Hack Squats, Leg Presses, Leg Extensions, Leg Curls and Lunges are the standard, proven exercises, and 12-20 sets constitute an adequate workout.

The "women's" exercises recommended by beauty experts are time-consuming and less effective. Those hundreds of doggy kicks and leg flings do not give deep muscle stimulation and can overwork joints and connective tissue.

Weight training is the most efficient method of firming, shaping and building muscles in the legs. Don't worry about developing huge legs. Large, bulky legs on women usually are due to thick subcutaneous fat. A bodybuilder's legs may look large onstage when oiled and flexed, but in reality they may be as small as 19" or 20" at the largest point.

Though a female bodybuilder may lose sufficient fat from her torso during a diet, fat may remain on her legs or hip area. It is so frustrating! Our female hormones cause us to have more fat and fluid retention. We have more fat cells, especially in the area from the waist to the knees.

Women often believe that fasting or radical dieting alone is effective in losing weight. You will lose weight this way, but only half of what you lose will be fat; the other half will be muscle. During severe dieting, the body, not certain when it will be fed again, attempts to hoard fat for future use, turning to muscle sources for energy. During a fast or a very restrictive diet, you might actually lose more muscle than fat. The result can be very poor muscle tone, plus an unattractive, soft appearance.

To ensure that you burn fat without burning muscle, you should make moderate changes in your diet. Initially, a reduction of 100-300 calories daily is sufficient. As time goes on, you should continue to reduce the calories provided by fat and refined carbohydrates. But don't eat less than 1,000 calories daily or create a deficit of more than 50% of your total daily caloric needs. If you do, you will surely lose muscle.

Fat loss is best accomplished by exercise, plus a moderate diet. Your body burns fat as fuel when you engage in low-intensity or moderate exercise for a prolonged period of time. On the other hand, during highly intense anaerobic exercise, fat isn't the principal fuel burned. The body utilizes glucose or glycogen (stored glucose in the liver and muscles) and protein. Therefore, aerobic exercise, such as dancing, skating, circuit weight training, brisk walking, jogging, cycling and swimming, is best for fat reduction.

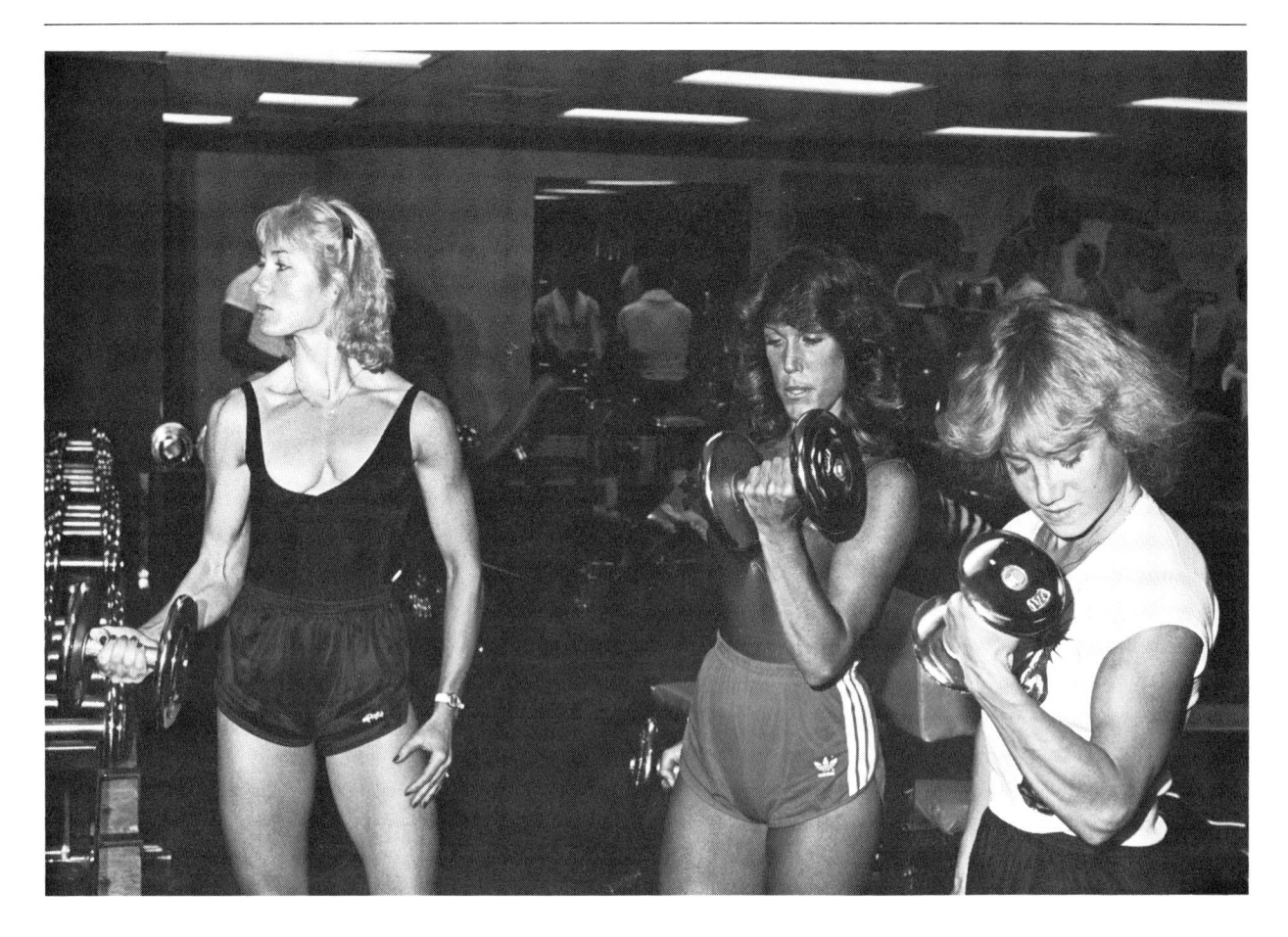

Weight training increases your lean muscle mass, making you firmer and more shapely. Adding muscle can speed up your calorie expenditures because muscle burns more calories per pound than do fat and connective tissue. But do not rely on weight training (unless you do it in circuit fashion) to aid considerably in fat loss. It is crucial for women to combine weight training with daily aerobic exercise for best results.

Excess subcutaneous fat is a by-product of being female, but you can conquer it. By combining added muscle with proper diet and aerobic exercise, any woman can be firmer, more shapely, and fit for life!□

Workouts Energize Every Cell in Your Body

by John Howell

Why exercise? Sure, exercise feels good and every Tom, Dick and Jane worth an Olympic bar will tell you it's good for you, but why? What happens to your body during and after exercise? A brief review of exercise physiology suggests a half dozen or so major physiological changes that result directly from exercise—changes that occur in the respiratory, circulatory, muscular, skeletal and nervous systems. In listing these changes, a logical starting place is the heart and circulatory system, since this system ultimately touches every one of the 75 trillion cells in your body.

The heart has one job to do. Pump blood. This is the most important job in the body, for if the heart malfunctions, this marvelous piece of machinery that we call a human being ceases to be. Exercise can't prevent heart malfunction, but it can minimize the chances of its occurrence. Exercise makes the heart muscle grow stronger, which increases its effectiveness as a pump. This means that the heart doesn't have to pump as often (i.e., a slower pulse rate) to get the job done. The heart then has a longer period between beats in which to rest. And since the heart muscle contracts during every beat for an entire lifetime, the only time it gets to rest is between beats. So a stronger heart gets to rest more often.

During exercise, the muscles need more oxygen. This means the lungs need more oxygen to put into the blood, which carries the oxygen to the muscles. During heavy exercise, the lungs are called upon to put up to 20 times as much oxygen into the blood as normal, and the blood flow to the muscles can also increase as much as 20 times normal.

Where does all this extra oxygen come from? The owner of the body being exercised breathes harder and faster. The harder, faster breathing is thought to be caused in part by stimulation of nerve receptors in the joints during joint movement. This is particularly true of aerobic exercise. The bodybuilder controls and coordinates his breathing with each rep. Think back to your early instruction in pumping iron: "Exhale forcefully during the power half of the rep," "Blow the weights away from you," etc.

As more oxygenated blood flows into the muscle, the muscle hypertropies (grows larger) and pumps up. What a fantastic feeling that pump is! Arnold Schwarzenegger calls it orgasmic. In the long run it builds larger, stronger muscles. And the increased blood flow makes the muscles healthier.

What about the bones? Muscles attach to bones, and a muscle's major job is to pull the bones on each end of it closer together. Think about it: When your bicep contracts, it causes your forearm to approach your shoulder. So as

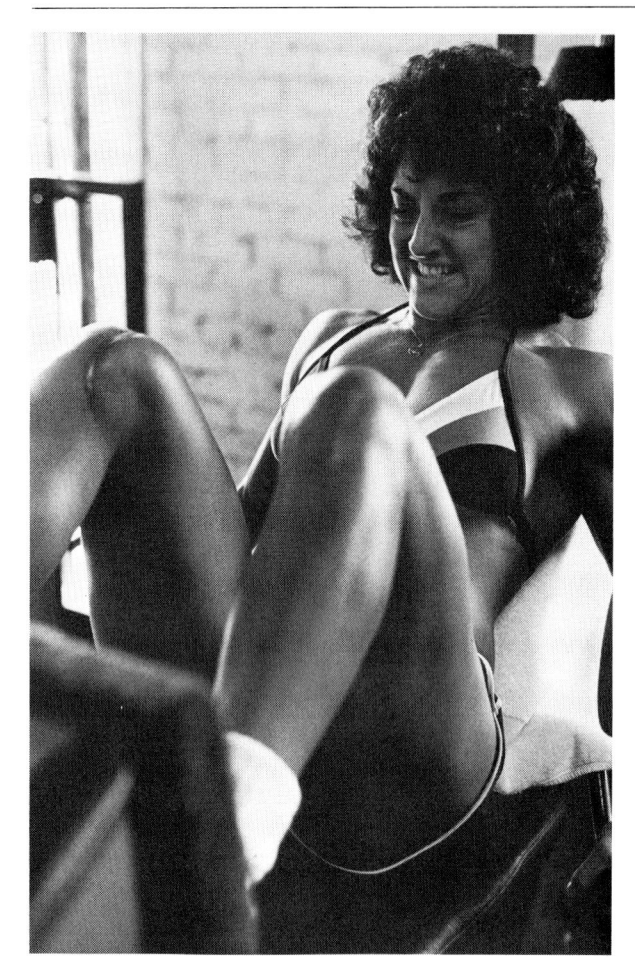

Laura Combes pushing hard.

muscles get stronger as a result of exercise, bones had better get stronger, too. Otherwise, they couldn't sustain the increased force of contraction. And that is just what happens. More calcium is deposited in the bones to make them stronger. Calcium deposition in bone involves a host of factors, including hormones, vitamins and other minerals.

The nervous system affects and is affected by exercising too. The nervous system controls everything that happens in the body. If the heart is becoming more efficient, and the lungs are breathing faster and harder, and the muscles are hypertrophying, and the bones are getting stronger, you can bet the nervous system isn't sitting idle. It's monitoring activity, making adjustments, regulating, shifting physiological emphasis to the bodypart being worked and generally staying in touch with everything. The nervous system directly benefits from exercise too, through improvement of the brain-to-muscle nerve pathways, a change which allows for more precise muscle control.

Of prime interest to the bodybuilder is the effect of exercise on the muscles themselves. Obviously, they grow bigger and stronger. But there are other benefits as well. The muscle fibers enjoy an increase in nutrient supply, due partly to the increased flow of nutrient-rich blood created by the demand of the muscle's hard work. The resting tone of the muscle improves also, although this is mainly the result of improved nerve activity.

There are two things to remember when exercising muscles for strength and bodybuilding purposes. The first is that weak muscular activity, even for long periods of time, doesn't produce muscular hypertrophy (increased size). Actually, no hypertrophy occurs unless the muscle contracts to at least 75% of its maximum. The second point to remember is what physiologists call the staircase effect, or treppe. When a muscle first begins to work after a period of rest, its initial strength may be as little as half what it will be later in the workout. This is the basis for lifting weights in sets. Everyone who has ever lifted weights knows that strength increases with each set until fatigue sets in.

These two things point to the fact that progressively increasing resistance (in other words, progressively heavier weights and increased muscular work) over a period of time is the only way to develop that elusive great physique.

One final point about exercise physiology: the relationship between exercise and stress. Exercise is a stress to the body, but a good stress. Hans Selye, MD, the father of stress research, calls this eustress. But exercise can also cause bad stress, or distress. If you have a lot going on in your life, exercise can add to everything else and finally become the straw that breaks the camel's back—distress. The exercising body has enough to handle. Don't overstress it.

As to "Why exercise?", the benefits are phenomenal. A stronger, more efficient heart; a well-developed relationship between breathing and circulation; increased size and strength of muscles and the bones they attach to; better brain-to-muscle coordination; and the introduction of a positive stress. In short, a well-exercised body is a better-functioning body.□

How Well Do Women Adapt to Exercise?

by Armand Tanny

Women's adaptation to exercise is one of the new frontiers in the field of exercise physiology. Women's real physical potential is still relatively unknown because in the past women weren't encouraged to develop their physical skills fully. In physiology research, recorded responses are not significant enough until the subject begins to exercise heavily, and most women simply didn't train hard enough to cause an adaptive response by the body, says exercise physiologist Christine Wells, Ph.D. Consequently, much of the existing research on female athletes may be of limited value, states Wells, a member of the American College of Sports Medicine.

Today, however, women are participating in high-stress sports and are responding to their greater physical workloads with results that compare favorably with those of men. Although much more research must be done, some interesting findings have already emerged. Wells, who is noted for her research on the differences between male and female tolerance to exercise and physical stress, has found that a person's fitness level, rather than sex, determines his or her ability to tolerate a hot environment. Also, structural similarities—not gender—determine comparable performance: elite male and female runners, for instance, had low bodyfat, were slight of build and had large aerobic capacities.

Another finding is that, in female athletes, cell walls may become fragile due to iron depletion during certain periods of the menstrual cycle. This causes nosebleeds or rupture of small blood vessels. Wells' research, conducted at the University of Iowa, suggests that iron loss may be the result of cell damage caused by the repetitive pounding of the feet during running.

Wells asks some interesting questions about this finding. Does it mean that women who run are more susceptible to cell damage or iron loss? Is it correct to assume that women are prone to anemia due to blood loss during menstruation? Do women who don't menstruate have a competitive advantage?

Exercise physiologists concede that high-intensity training of any kind, including bodybuilding, results in blood-cell damage. Training too hard in the early phases of a program can result in anemia. Normally, in the process of adaptation, the cells are replaced. But are they replaced sufficiently to support a subsequent higher level of exercise stress?

Wells is skeptical of the benefits of exercising at many health spas: "(Women) are going into these places and are being pounded, massaged, overheated and generally abused. They're given weird pills and diets to follow. It's terrible. When you look at what they call aerobics, you discover that all it involves is calisthenics done in time to music.

"We'd like to work with them to develop a curriculum, some courses in basic physiology, exercise and anatomy, and possibly give some workshops for their instructors. I'd like to see more physical educators—those with a background in sports physiology or kinesiology who could conduct a proper fitness class—working in spas. It would help upgrade the industry." ("Christine Wells: Asking the Right Questions," by Jim Ferstle, *The Physician and Sportsmedicine*, July 1982.)

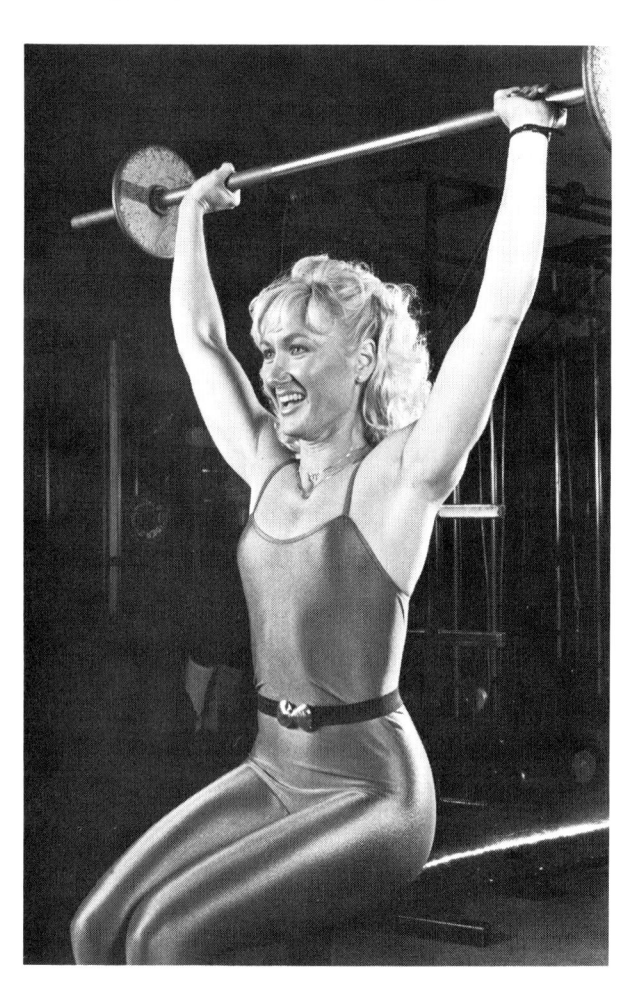

Not enough women want to work in exercise physiology, Wells says. Despite federal prohibition of sex discrimination, there are few female role models in this area. But for women interested in an exciting, challenging, new field, this is it!

Getting the Most from Your Health Club

by Kristine Randal and Joy Grau

Millions of people are flocking to health clubs to get fit and firm—50 million Americans will exercise today—but many are overlooking some valuable benefits their clubs offer. Here are tips to help you discover all the programs, equipment, services and advice your club provides, so you can get the most from your membership, RIGHT NOW.

Investigate Programs and Activities

Believe it or not, there's more going on in your health club than weightlifting, aerobics and stretching. Although incorporating these three exercise programs into your weekly workout is effective, this routine will eventually lose its newness. Spice up your visits to the gym by adding specialty classes like gymnastics, self-defense, pool exercises, yoga or even belly dancing. You'll not only have fun, but perhaps discover a new hobby, talent or career. Who knows, you might end up as the exotic belly dancer at a popular Moroccan restaurant.

Don't overlook personal services. After a grueling workout reward yourself with a trip to the jacuzzi or steam room, followed by a refreshing plunge in the pool. Or better yet, if your club offers it, indulge yourself in a Swedish-style massage, herbal facial or manicure.

Read the newsletters and posters scattered about your club to learn about holistic health care, bodybuilding seminars and diet through behavior modification. Take advantage of body composition results from testing services that periodically visit major health facilities. Perhaps that weight you've been worrying about is more muscle than fat. If so, then you simply may have a job of toning to do. Many educational programs offer special discounts to club members.

If your club is limited in its activities, voice your suggestions. Maybe your club wasn't aware of the intense interest in pregnancy exercise classes. You should also scan the bulletin board, which is always jam-packed with useful information.

Acquaint Yourself with Equipment and Facilities

At first glance, the vast array of complicated looking pulleys, machines and heavy weights is not only impressive, but rather intimidating as well! Take the challenge and turn these cold-chromed designs into your closest friends by learning how the equipment works. Ask the instructor about any apparatus not familiar to you. If you see another member performing an unusual exercise, ask him or her about it. It's imperative to learn not only the proper movements of the equipment, but also what they

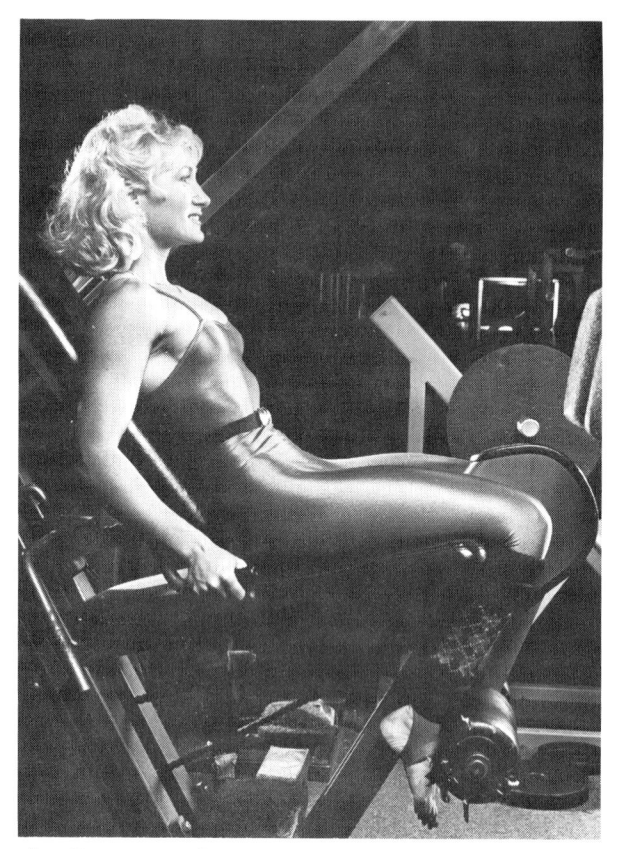

Claudia Cornwell Wilbourn works her thighs on a Nautilus Leg Extension machine.

do for your body and which muscle groups are affected.

As your knowledge of the equipment grows, you'll be able to add variety to your workouts. By mixing and matching cables, free weights and machines, you'll get the results you're after. For example, your program may call for Bent Rowing. But if the pulley isn't available or if you want a change, substitute Wide-Grip Chins, Seated Rows or barbells.

Once familiar with the exercise equipment, check out other facilities, such as that interesting contraption in the corner, the rock steam bath or therapeutic whirlpool.

Use All Training Aids Efficiently

After you become acquainted with the facilities and equipment, your next step is learning to use them efficiently. There is a right way and wrong way to perform exercises. Here are some tips for doing them right:

1. Always use the proper movement of the exercise. This goes hand in hand with using the correct amount of weight (not too light as to offer little resistance, nor too heavy, prompting undue strain). For instance, when attempting Bench Presses with an overly weighted barbell,

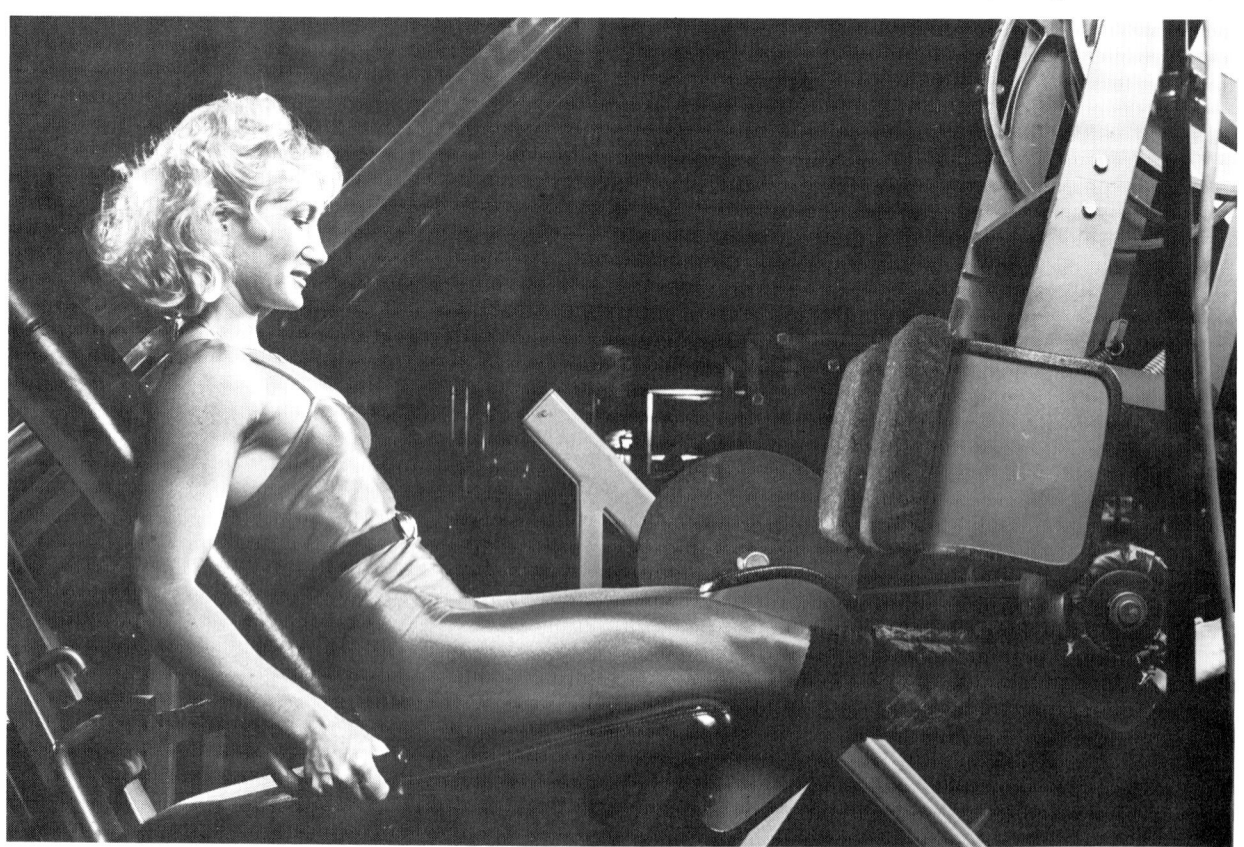

you might be forced to cheat. In this case you'll try to compensate by arching your back. This will cause you to miss the intended effect on the arms, shoulders and chest. You'll also miss the benefits of carrying the weight through its full range of motion.

2. On various exercises, place the hands so the weight will be handled most efficiently for the muscle group being emphasized. When doing Triceps French Presses, for example, the hands should be fairly close together for a more concentrated effect.

3. Your stance can have a bearing on the precise muscle affected. For example, pointing your toes in or out can change the focus of a calf exercise. During Sit-Up movements, bent knees can prevent minor back injuries. In the end, your stance or position should contribute to both the safety and efficiency of an exercise.

4. When using machines, make sure seats and belts are adjusted to fit you properly.

The best use of facilities includes combining activities to compliment each other: a warm-up in the stretching class—a workout in the weight or exercise room—a few minutes in the sauna—ending with a dip in the pool. By the time you've finished showering, you'll feel cleansed, strong and invigorated.

Become Socially Involved

Who knows . . . maybe the woman doing heavy Squats is a scuba diving or snow skiing instructor! By being friendly to her you may soon find yourself skiing down a powdery slope or diving for a lobster dinner off some enchanting island. It's easy to make friends. Simply compliment others when they turn up with an attractive striped leotard or a new tan. Ask another her secret for her slender waist. If familiar members have lost weight recently or firmed up their triceps, break the ice and let them know you've noticed. You'll be introducing yourself to new friends, hobbies and experiences. Your club will become a place to hone both body and social skills.

Make the Most of Your Workout Time

While you want to make friends, remember that you paid money to improve your body. Making friends is one thing, but breaking up the rhythm of your workouts by talking too long is another. Instead, meet friends in the sauna, jacuzzi or juice bar—after your training.

Where do you spend most of your club time—in the sauna or in aerobics class? Make the most of your club visit by structuring your time properly. I think of my stretching session as an appetizer. It prepares my body for the main course—aerobics or weightlifting, where I spend most of my time, burning calories and reaping cardiovascular benefits. For dessert, I treat myself to a sauna or jacuzzi.

To help you plan your physically fit menu, ask an instructor for advice. Tell her your physical goals, and stick to the plan the two of you create. If you want to gain weight or reshape your body, emphasize resistance training. If you'd like to lose weight and tone up, stress aerobics and diet. In any case, a balanced weekly program of aerobics, weightlifting and stretching will render optimum results.

Go to the gym with a plan for each workout. Know what bodypart you're going to work, the exercises you'll perform, and in what order you'll do them. With a plan, you won't be wasting time and can maintain a more consistent training pace. But keep in mind that your workout plan is only a plan. You created it—you can change it. It should give you a firm idea of what you're going to do, but not be so inflexible as to prevent you from adding a new exercise, deleting a set or changing the order.

Ask the staff what they think are the best training hours. Some health facilities open up as early as six in the morning and close around nine in the evening, or even later. Ask yourself whether you're a morning or evening person, and schedule your workouts accordingly. If your club is close to work, consider exercising during your lunch hour.

Make the most of your workout time by being consistent. Attend the gym on a regular basis, whether you feel like it or not! (You'll be glad you did.)

Take Advantage of Your Club's Attractions and Specials

Although some people feel they're well in tune with what their club has to offer, further investigation may turn up a few surprises. Did you know about that membership drive starting next month? Or about the two-for-one special? Or the gym bag that's being offered for new referrals? Check into such options and see how you can benefit. Ask the staff to keep you informed concerning new classes, new membership benefits and club-sponsored events.

Before vacationing, get an extension on your membership. Inform your club that you'll be gone so that you won't be charged for time you missed. Ask about affiliated clubs in the cities you'll visit, and use them.

Get to Know Instructors and Staff

As already mentioned, the staff at your gym is a wonderful resource. All instructors are interested in the progress of individual club members. However, becoming better acquainted with a staff member will ensure a closer monitoring of your personal program. It only stands to reason that if you take more interest in what your instructor does, she'll take more interest in what you do.

Sticking to your fitness program will be more pleasurable if you know someone on the staff cares about you. The better the employees of your health club know you, the more they're able to sense when you need instruction, critique and encouragement. We all do our best "with a little help from our friends."

If you already are a health-club member, start investigating these ideas today. If you're still shopping, use these considerations as a guide.

Remember, if you know you're getting the most from your health club, you'll get the most from your body!

Body Sculpture and Muscularity:
Two Separate Events for Women?

by Joe Weider (Pro) and Sheila Herman (Con)

Pro: Reward Both Physiques

The debate rages. Do we reward the most muscular woman or the one who's sleek and aesthetic-looking? Why not split a contest into two parts and end the bickering?

After all, there seem to be two types of female physiques. Some women can muscle up almost as much as men. They get big and ripped at the same time. A lot of effort goes into that achievement and it should be rewarded. But some women will never look like that, no matter how hard they train. They just don't have the same chemistry. The second physique is more feline, slimmer. Two distinct builds—each deserves to win.

Both realize their potential in ways that result in two different body shapes. But a stocky, muscular woman can't be compared to a woman who has a refined, slender build.

It's not like the men. Male bodybuilders have comparable physiques. They possess wide shoulders and narrow hips. (Not all women have this V-shape by virtue of their skeletal frame.) Men strive for balanced maximum muscle size and are able to cause muscle hypertrophy simply because they *are* men. Many women can't pack on the thick, dense musculature that men do. Women are repeatedly reassured: because you lack sufficient quantities of male hormone, you won't look like Arnold Schwarzenegger if you lift weights.

Con: Bodybuilding is Both!

Creating two contests hedges the issue. What people want is a clear direction in the sport, and a division at this time won't provide it. To some, the only choices are between woman-bodybuilders-as-sex-kitten or as muscle-bound freak.

It's easy to see how this controversy got started. In less than a year, we went from Miss Bikini to Ms. Biceps. No wonder heads are spinning!

But that whirlwind transformation doesn't mean this is an either/or choice, a pick-one-or-the-other (or even a pick-both-to-make-everybody-happy) situation. It just represents a natural oscillation like a pendulum set in motion. The pendulum swings to both sides until it settles, and where it settles is where all things that succeed eventually land. Right in the center.

In this case, the middle ground is a balance of aesthetics and muscles. Since the sport is new, the pendulum is still swinging. For now, at least, there really do seem to be two different female physiques.

But two separate events in one contest at this time would be a big mistake. It would sever the natural evolution of women's bodybuilding. This ersatz solution wouldn't solve the problem and would create new ones.

The trouble with splitting up the contests is that you're still stuck with the same old

Pro: Reward Both Physiques (Continued)

There are exceptions, of course. Some women are capable of becoming massive, and they seem to overshadow their slighter sisters. Why penalize one or the other type when both have trained just as strenuously?

There is a wide range of different body shapes among female bodybuilders. Some women are broad-shouldered and narrow-hipped, while others have the petite, traditionally feminine build tailored with muscle without being overpowering. Consider the contrast between Pillow and Candy Csencsits. Naturally, this range of female physiques creates a problem.

In one contest we could have the two categories. This will satisfy the beefcake-hungry crowd that's interested only in densely muscled women. This will also satisfy the general public, which sees bodybuilding as a sport in which a slight woman who trains to improve her appearance can win.

Each faction has a following. After every contest, there are angry outbursts from both sides. If a shapely muscular woman loses, she

Con: Bodybuilding is Both! (Continued)

question: What's the judging criteria? For body sculpture, do you use the traditional guidelines, i.e., pretty face, generous bust, wasp waist, voluptuous hips, long legs, etc.? What are you looking for in terms of muscularity—16-inch biceps, cross-striated quadriceps, abdominals like the Grand Canyon?

If we go that route, we can replace the three-round IFBB point system with a tape measure for the Hulkettes and hold a hand over the heads of the Glamourites and measure crowd applause! Sort of gets away from the original idea of the sport, doesn't it?

Fact is, the problem of choosing one quality over the other is solving itself. Sure, some women are still coming into contests relying more on their natural gifts—usually the ones mistakenly associated with symmetry—than on their muscularity. Still other women are stronger in the muscle department than they are in beauty.

But bodybuilding is both: beauty and brawn. Always has been, always will be. Muscular

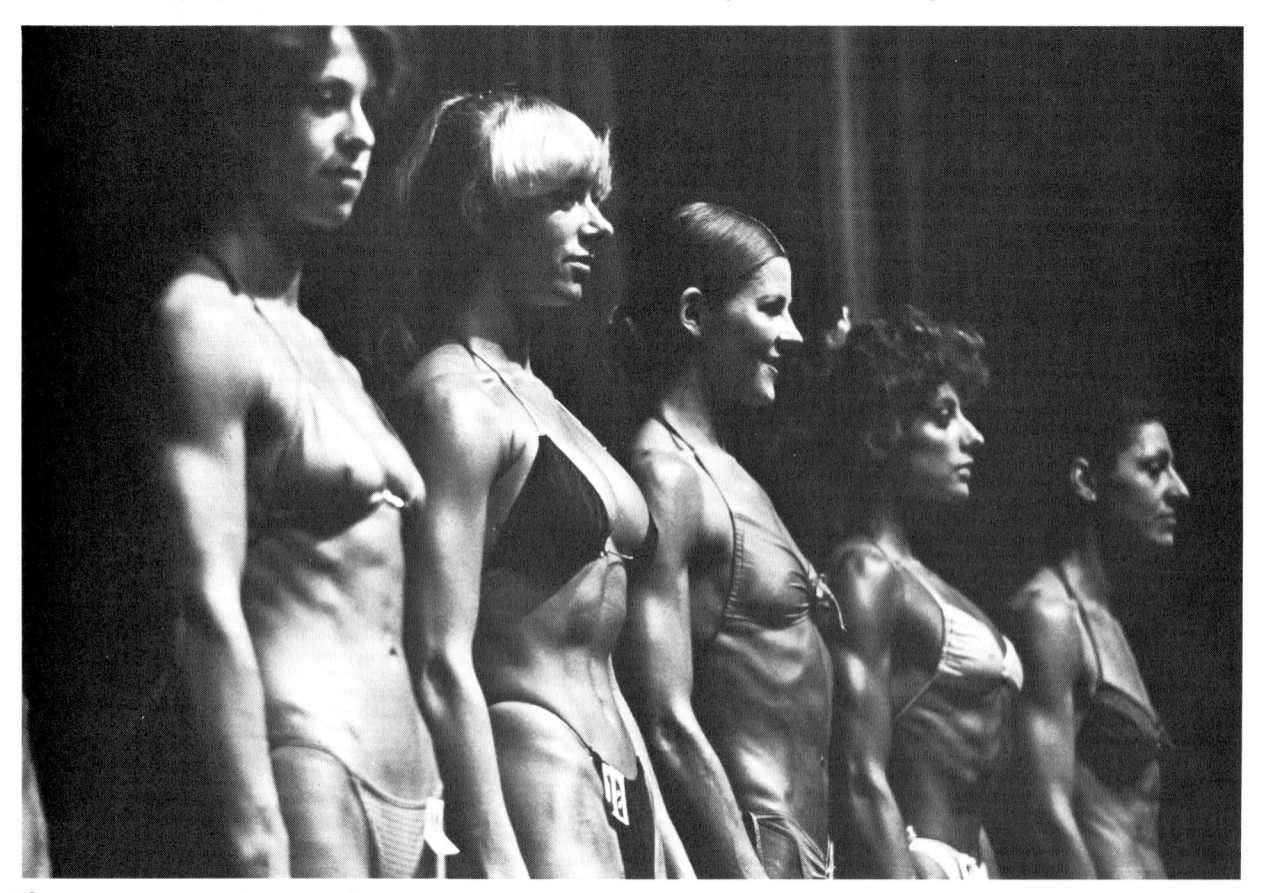

The 1981 European Championship.

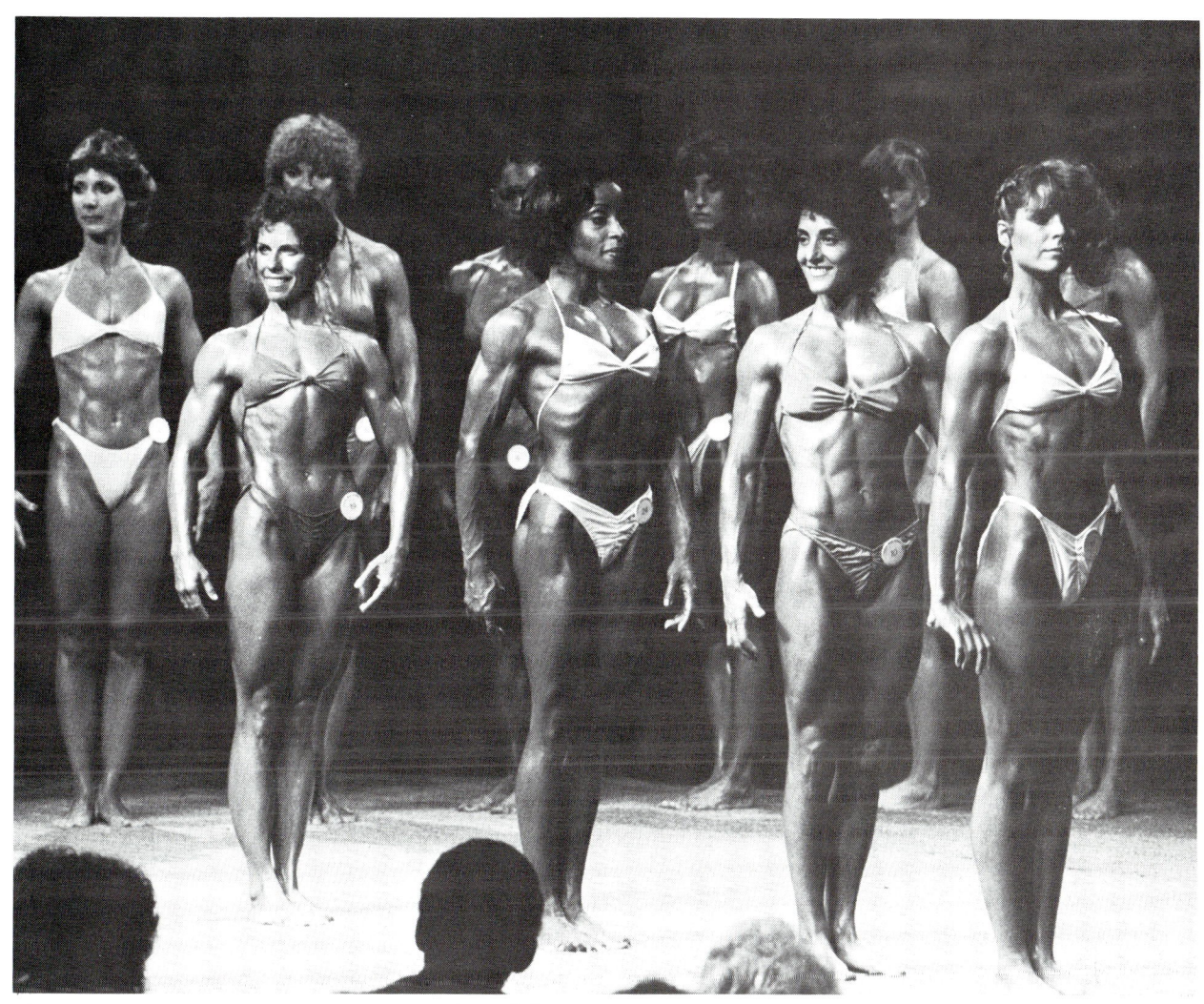

The 1982 Miss Olympia. Front four, from left to right, are Lynn Conkwright, Carla Dunlap, Laura Combes, and Candy Csencsits.

Pro: Reward Both Physiques (Continued)

feels cheated. Her hours in the gym seem unappreciated. Yet when a well-developed, symmetrical woman loses to a very muscular one, the former might ask herself, Do I have to look like *that* to win?

To some women, getting ultra ripped or having 14-inch arms is impossible and in some cases undesirable. Truth is, women need both role models. In this day and age being strong, muscular and shapely appeals to most women. There is even an attraction to macha—the female equivalent of macho. Remember, a woman's specific genetic inheritance and basic structure and shape determine how her body develops through weight training.

There are two general ways a woman

Con: Bodybuilding is Both! (Continued)

development is a prerequisite, but having good looks never hurt a man and there's no reason to expect anything different with a woman.

The trouble with even thinking in terms of separating the contest is that if a woman feels that she'll be rewarded more for either sculpture or muscularity then she's likely to pursue whichever comes easier for her. A woman who's gotten by on her looks all her life might be reluctant to admit that she needs to train intensely. Likewise, a woman who gets attention by being muscular may not aim for anything but sheer size.

It's human to shun the tasks that are more difficult. In bodybuilding, one must own up to her flaws and try to eradicate them. We know

Pro: Reward Both Physiques (Continued)

bodybuilder can look. Which fits her personality and physical potential should be a winning look. Both the very muscular woman and the slighter woman can be highly aesthetic.

As we grow in experience, the two events could possibly be combined, just as it has been in men's bodybuilding. Meanwhile, we can encourage women with both bodytypes to train hard and enter the contests, thus swelling our ranks. We should avoid too much controversy, which could tear our sport apart during this developmental stage.

Why let disagreement create losers when there is a way for everyone to win?

Con: Bodybuilding is Both! (Continued)

from watching the men that this process takes a long time—much longer than women's bodybuilding has been around.

In time, what seems to be two distinct physiques will turn out to be the same animal, namely a female bodybuilder. For now, contest results are confusing and the direction of the sport is not apparent to the casual observer.

To the learned student of all things bodybuilding, it's undeniable. You've got to have both qualities to win. Without the clay of body sculpture—muscles—the artist cannot complete her task.

There's room for short-term rewards in the present system. Most Muscular and Most Symmetrical trophies can be awarded. Ideally, the woman who wins should be the closest to both.

Two separate contests at this point would prevent that ideal from ever happening.

The Will to Win!

by Laura Combes

The human mind, if correctly utilized, is phenomenally powerful. It has sent men to the moon, fostered great civilizations and developed a generation of bodybuilders that would have blown the minds of iron game cognoscenti only a decade or two ago.

Yes, ladies, you have within yourselves a power that can turn you into a superwoman if you can learn how to use it. But how? In this article I will tell you how, and then you can begin to achieve your personal bodybuilding goals.

At a seminar recently an aspiring woman bodybuilder asked me how much of my success in the sport could be attributed to my mental approach. I told her 100%. I can—and have—dieted and trained optimally for a competition but not appeared onstage in peak condition, because my mind wasn't fully into it. Unless the mind triggers the ability to improve and peak, all the training and strict dieting in the world will be a complete waste.

If you don't have the will to win, you simply will be unable to endure the grueling training and strict diet necessary to win a high-level bodybuilding title. I've been a winner in bodybuilding and several other sports, and I like the feeling. I know that when I am doing absolutely everything I can in my workouts and am strictly adhering to my precontest diet, I will win.

Two months before I won the American Championship in September 1980 I wrote in my training diary, "If you want to become the American Champion you must reach deep within yourself to bring out that will to win that can only come from yourself. You must deny yourself lesser desires and pleasures and strive for what is most important to you. With these things in mind, you alone can determine your fate. With these things accomplished, the victory will be yours and yours alone."

I did reach deep enough for that special will to win. As I trained to win the America, I knew that no one in her right mind would have pushed as hard as I did, so I was sure I would win. To reach my goal, I willingly tortured myself in the gym each day.

Bodybuilding is an exacting taskmistress. It doesn't allow people with weak wills to win. There is no room among the sport's great champions for anyone without a burning desire to succeed against all odds, to strive with the fabled last ounce of courage to reach a cherished goal.

The effort of properly preparing to win a contest just isn't worth it unless you actually do win. It takes all my will-power, self-discipline, desire and courage to prepare to win, and it's silly to make such an investment merely to take home a second- or third-place trophy. I totally focus on an upcoming competition, sacrificing

26 BODYBUILDING AND CONDITIONING FOR WOMEN

my social life—and everything else that ordinary women consider important—to appear at my best onstage.

If you're incapable of putting forth your best effort, you're better off staying out of competition until you *are* capable. You might place fairly well in a contest with less than 100% effort, but you won't win.

So developing the will to win—the will to achieve greatness—is the first step. Without it, you will be condemned to the ranks of also-rans and might-have-beens. Do you want more than anything else in life to succeed as a bodybuilder? If you do, you're on your way.

Next, you must set goals in your bodybuilding preparations. Bodybuilding goals come in two varieties, long- and short-range. A long-range goal is the ultimate degree of physical conditioning you plan to reach. Short-range goals are segments of that long-range goal, segments that seem more easily reachable than the pie-in-the-sky goal.

In bodybuilding training, the more weight you use in the Bench Press, the more muscular your pectorals and deltoids will become. Say you can now do 6 reps in the Bench Press with 100 pounds, it's difficult to conceptualize doing 6 reps with 100 pounds. Let's say, however, that you wish over a two-year period to work up to using 150 pounds for your Benches. Committing yourself to achieving this is a long-range goal.

To add 50 pounds to your Bench Press in two years, you will need to add only 2½ pounds each month. This 2½ pounds is an achievable short-range goal, and achieving a series of such goals will inevitably bring you to your long-range goal of boosting your Bench Press to 150 pounds. You can imagine how much more impressive your upper body will be by the time you actually handle this poundage.

Imagining how you will look is your next step to establishing a good mental approach to bodybuilding. When I first committed myself to the sport, I established a mental image of how I wanted to eventually look. And over the years, despite many assaults by judges and other bodybuilding officials on it, I have maintained that same image.

During the past year, a number of photos of me with a softer appearance have been published in *Muscle & Fitness*, leading some of my fans to think that I have compromised my concept of physical perfection. Actually, however, I was just as hard when those photos were taken as I was onstage at a competition.

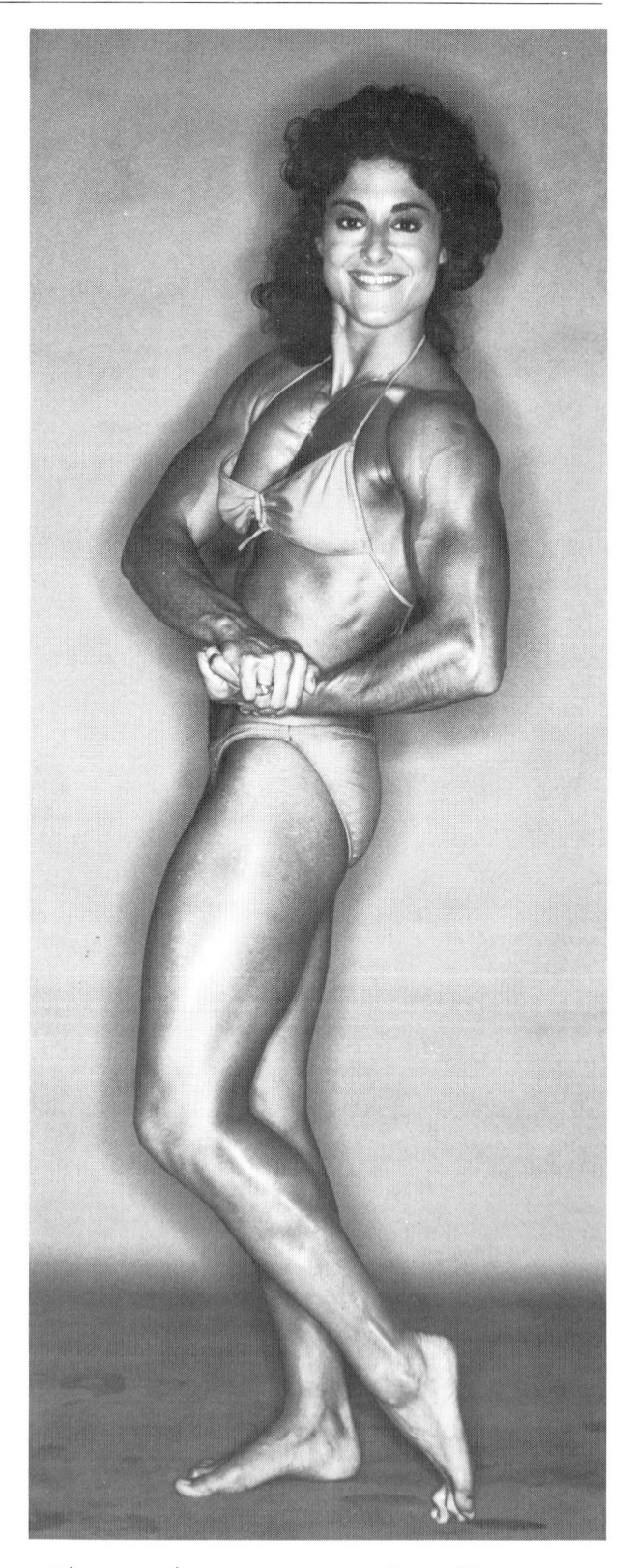

Photographs can create a variety of images. Lighting, especially in bodybuilding photography, creates the mood. And in these newer photos the lighting and camera lens made me look softer.

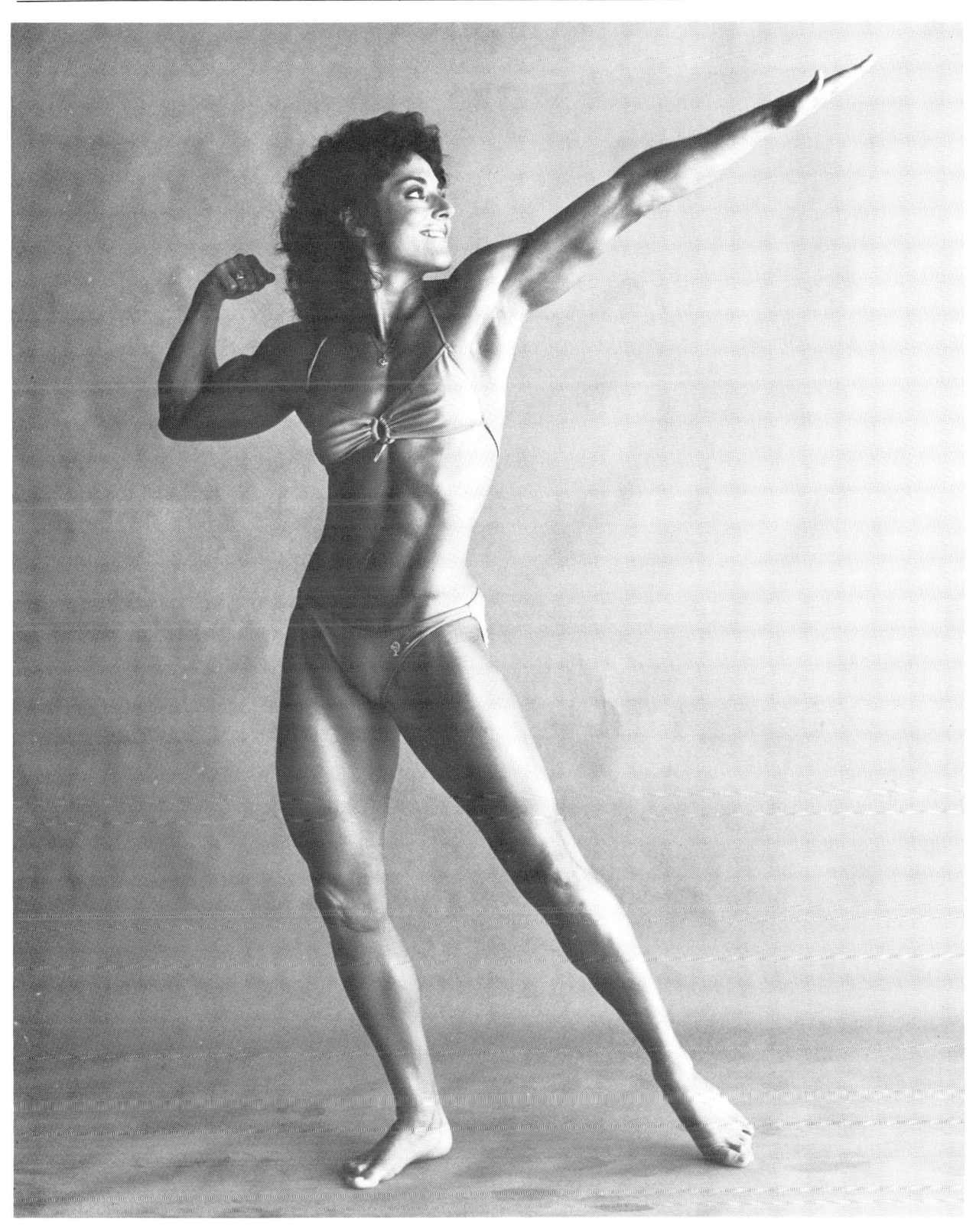

Femininity can be either soft or hard. My first love is to be as massive as possible and very muscular, but I'm not going to confine myself to that image. I want to achieve physical balance at the same time in order to achieve an aesthetic overall appearance. Women can and should have muscle mass and look muscular if they are going to call themselves bodybuilders.

Regardless of the route the judging of women's bodybuilding takes, I'm going to stick to my guns and come into a contest looking like *I* feel a female bodybuilder should look. Pressure from the public or bodybuilding officials won't dissuade me. I may change my appearance from the neck up (hairstyle and makeup), but from the neck down I will be a *bodybuilder*.

I'm not trying to influence you in choosing the type of body you'd like to attain. Femininity can be either soft or hard, and the choice is yours. Once you make it, however, stick to your guns. It doesn't matter what someone else likes, because you live with your body. Go for what *you* like.

As you develop your image of future physical perfection, make it as realistic as possible. When you close your eyes, see every detail of muscular development, every vein, every cut. Your image should be so vivid that it's like a film image projected on the inside of your eyelids.

Once you have this image firmly established, you can use it to program your subconscious mind to help you attain your goals. Once your subconscious mind is properly programmed, it can help you to avoid eating junk foods and missing workouts, and to be totally committed. Then bodybuilding becomes a joy rather than a burden.

Visualization is an operative form of what psychologists call "self-actualization." You've probably seen women who have dreamed for years about being a nurse or pilot or whatever, and they eventually reach their goals. They do so through self-actualization, or through an unconscious visualization process.

To consciously visualize, set aside about 20 minutes each night before you fall asleep. Simply lie relaxed and conjure up your image of physical perfection. Doing this regularly will efficiently program your mind. It's almost like creative daydreaming. Maybe this sounds simplistic to you, but it works for a bodybuilder or any other athlete.

The more you visualize, the better you will become at it. Eventually, you'll be able to feel what it's like in competition almost to the point where you can smell the oil on your body. You can even feel what it's like to win. When you get to this point, you're in.

At the America in 1980 I had visualized my victory so completely I couldn't wait to get onstage. I knew I was the best and this gave me a winner's body language. If you go to enough bodybuilding competitions, you'll see women with this body language, as well as women who look like losers the second they step onstage, even though they may have very good development.

Some champion bodybuilders periodically update their mental images over the years, but I've stuck with the same one. The only change has been in my physique as I come closer and closer to reaching this image. I look for improvements in my weaker areas as short-range goals, but I'm constantly after my pie-in-the-sky long-range goal, which is ultimately achieving the image I have set for myself.

My final mental bodybuilding technique is to ask myself motivational questions each day: Do you want to reach a new level of personal excellence? Do you want to go beyond what you've done before? Will you sacrifice to reach your goals?

You can't fool yourself when you ask these questions, because bodybuilding takes genuine commitment and effort. Unfortunately, many women bodybuilders lie to themselves. You know from looking at them that they're not doing what they say they are, because they'd look much better if they were. So you have to be honest with yourself. See your weak points and do something about them.

If you use the mental techniques I've outlined in this article, you can be a superwoman someday.□

Winning Takes More Than Muscle

by Sheila Herman

Every woman wants to win, but in any contest, only one woman can win. How does she do it? Simple—she doesn't lose! That is, she doesn't set herself up to lose by walking onstage looking like a loser.

Winning bodybuilding goes beyond muscle building. Being a winner means paying attention to *every* detail in physique presentation—attitude, posture, skin condition, posing suit, hair and more.

These details can make the difference between winning and losing.

Of course, having a good physique is most of the game in bodybuilding. But beyond training long and hard, beyond strict dieting, you can do more. When you step onstage, your attitude must signal, like a neon sign flashing over your head, "I'M A WINNER!"

The first thing the judges and audience notice is how you walk onstage. The best way to make your entrance is with a quiet, confident walk. Your steps should be bold strides. Never, *never* stomp. If you want to instantly create a negative impression, stomp across the stage like an elephant.

How you stand is also part of your image. Do you stand like a winner, or slouch like a loser? Do you keep your head up proudly, or are you checking your toenails? A winner keeps her eyes focused straight ahead. When standing relaxed, her feet, ankles and knees are together and her shoulders are pulled back at relaxed attention. A winner stands tall even if she's short. She demands recognition by the way she stands—and usually gets it.

Lynn Conkwright is a perfect example of good posture. Her stance isn't rigid or slouchy, but graceful and relaxed. All her bones are well aligned so she seems to stand straight effortlessly. To do the same, imagine each of your vertebrae stacked in a neat, unbending column. Proper posture always makes a good impression.

Here's a physiology question that relates to our subject: what's the biggest organ "in" your body? You're right if you answered "skin." There sure is a lot of it, and in bodybuilding almost all of it shows. It's a regular skin game. A suntan, a healthy appearance and taut skin are crucial.

A suntan is a must in our sport. Never mind that you don't tan easily or can't get out in the sun regularly. You can get around these problems. Buying your own sunlamp is smart. Or consider a tanning salon. If you are clever, like Debbie Trenholm, you can reduce your expenses. She persuaded a tanning salon to let her bask in their sunlamps for free.

Contestants know about all the instant tanning products on the market, but some of these individuals wonder if it's okay to use a fake tan

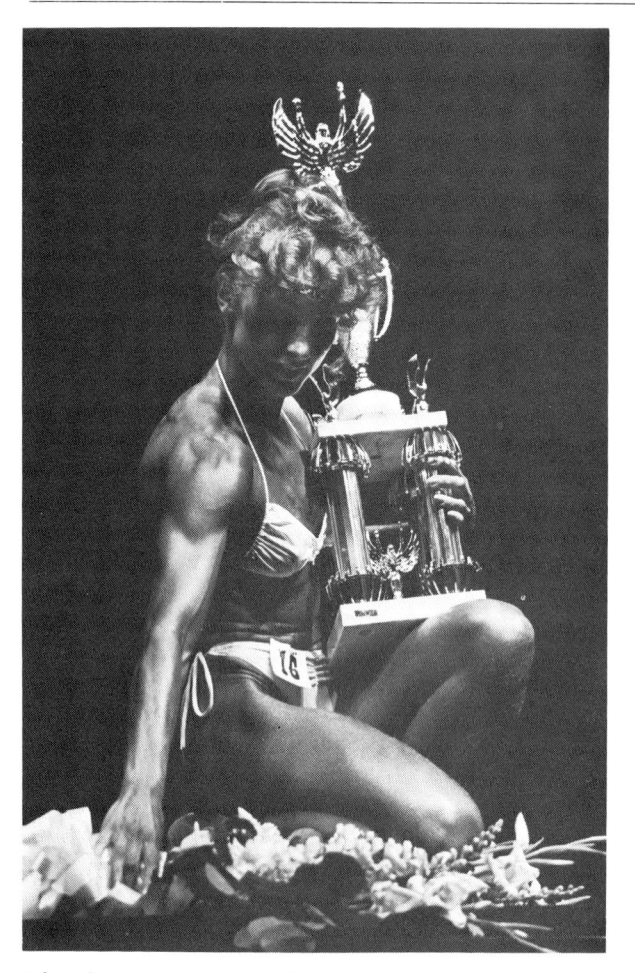

Kike Elomaa, winner of the 1981 European Championship.

loss. Varicose veins are also fairly common. But common or not, why allow them to show when it's perfectly legal to cover them? Likewise, being tanned disguises minor skin blemishes. If you have problem skin it is worthwhile to consult a dermatologist. In the meantime, head for the sun. Scars are considered a flaw. Plastic surgery to correct them may be too drastic; a tan is a sensible alternative. In the long run, a bodybuilder wants to have a natural, healthy glow without using tanning products. Tanning products should be only a short-term camouflage for pale or sallow skin.

Poor skin tone is another common flaw. Skin tone relates to the tightness of the skin. Most women have naturally taut skin, but some women sacrifice their skin's tautness in an effort to be lean. With women's bodybuilding in a state of flux, many women are relying heavily on dieting to achieve the lean, defined look. While diet is part of the game, too rapid a weight loss can have negative effects. One effect is a loss of skin tone. If a woman is losing weight faster than her skin can contract, her skin will sag. The solution is to lose more slowly, keeping pace with the skin's ability to adjust.

Enough on skin. Let's talk about what covers it—your posing suit. Almost every woman has

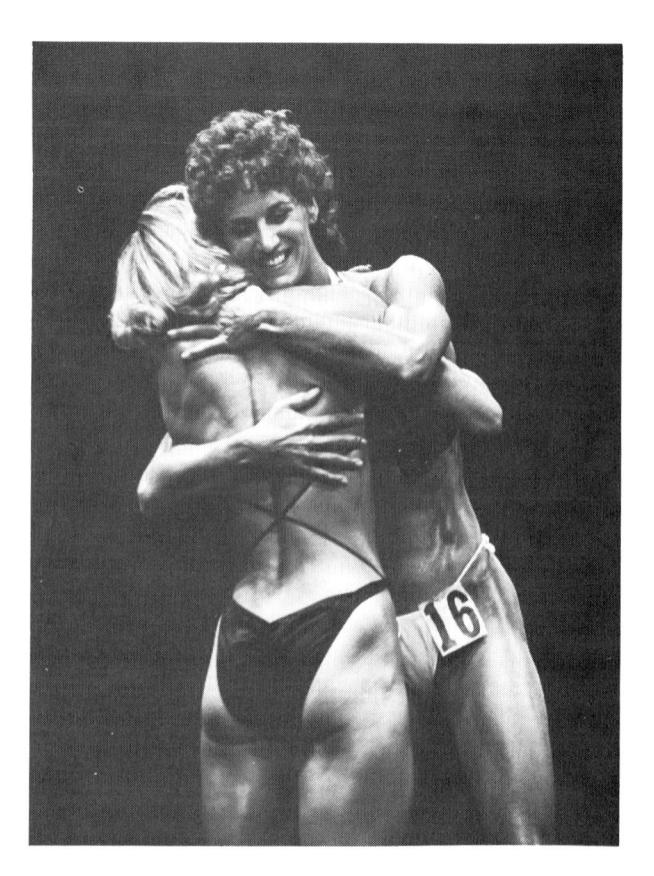

lotion. Yes, it's acceptable. The rules say tanning products are allowed if they are applied a day before the contest. Just make sure that you have experimented with several brands well ahead of time to find the one that works best for you. Several thin coats usually give the most natural look. Remember to wash the lotion off the palms of your hands. Tanned palms make your tan look phony.

Some people keep their tanning techniques secret. The magic concoction that made Lisa Elliott a dynamite bronze for the America is still a mystery. Although several contestants asked her, she wouldn't tell. Reasonably, you can expect an answer only from someone you aren't competing against, so find a *guy* whose color you like and ask him what he uses. (In any case, it's a great way to meet him.)

A tan creates a healthy, sunny appearance. It also hides stretch marks, varicose veins, minor skin blemishes and scars. Many women have stretch marks from childbearing or quick weight

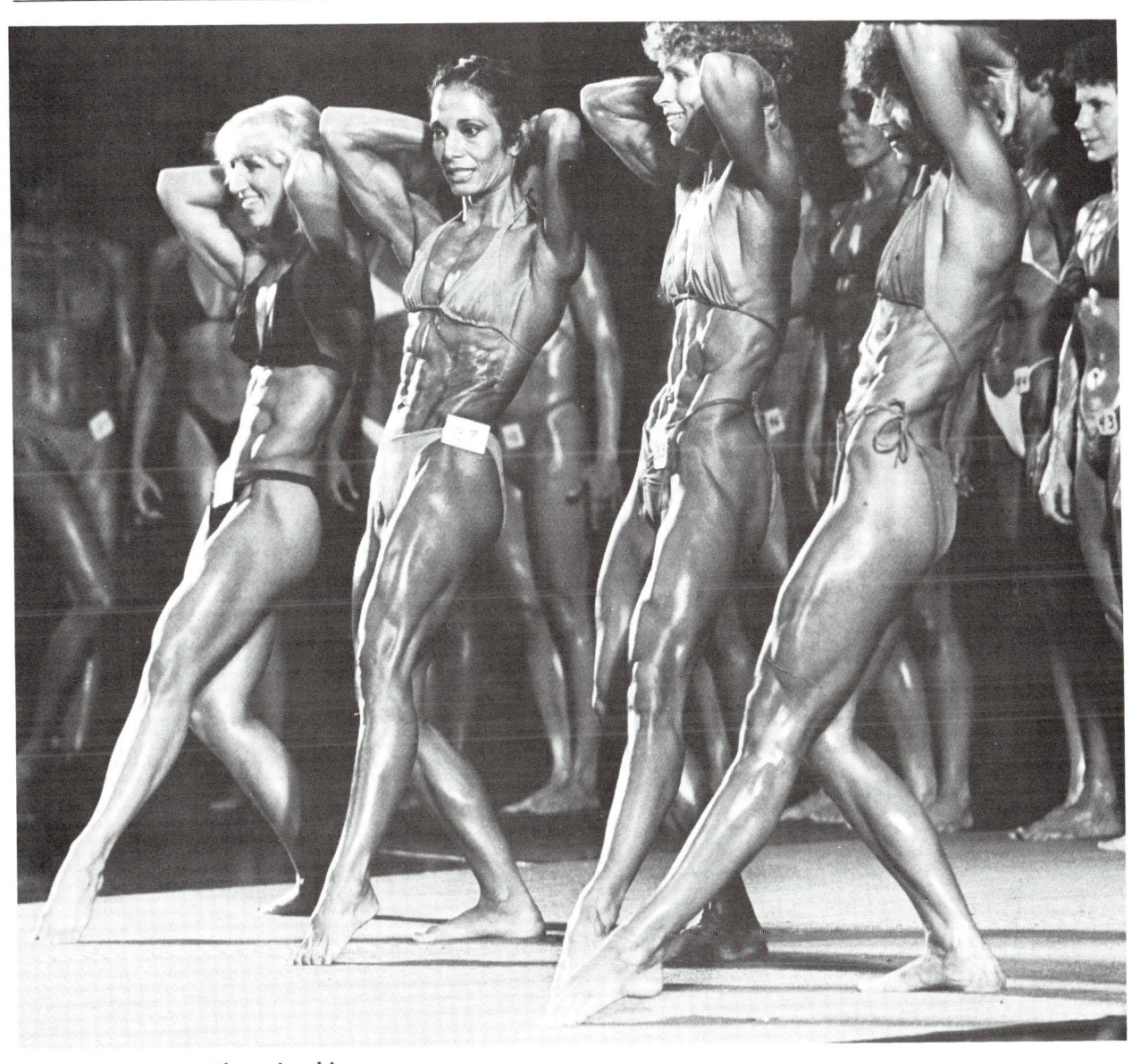

The 1982 American Championship.

had the experience of buying two bathing suits. One is a modeling bathing suit that you wear for sunbathing and lounging around the pool. It never gets wet. The other one is more practical—you wear it to actually go swimming. A posing suit has to be a combination of the two—both functional and flattering. A posing suit has to do a lot more than make you look sexy. It has to stay in place while you are raising your arms, lunging or doing your exotic back handspring into a front double biceps pose. You don't want the judges to be wondering, "Is her suit going to snap off?" (It has happened!) And stopping during your posing routine to adjust your suit can cost you points.

A posing suit has to stay in place, but also should be flattering, like the one Carla Dunlap wore to win the 1981 Ms. America contest. Chris Reed took a special pleasure in Carla's win. Instead of her usual blue suit, Carla wore a white posing suit Chris had loaned her. Chris is convinced that the different colored suit gave Carla the winning edge. Who will ever know how much of a difference it made? In any case, the right color and style of posing suit can help you look your best.

It shouldn't be necessary to mention shaving, but I have noticed some unshaven women in competition. Hairy legs were more apparent at the World Games last summer than at any other contest. Even if acceptable in Europe, hairy legs and armpits have no place in bodybuilding. You also should make sure pubic hair isn't peeking out of your posing suit.

Speaking of hair, let's talk about hairstyles. Although the rules require that hair be pulled off the back, it isn't necessary to wear a tight ponytail or bun. Many hairstyles are becoming and yet are within the guidelines. For short hair, a fluffy hairstyle like Deborah Diana's is great. Long hair can be softly pinned up, maintaining fullness and shape around the face for a feminine look. Or pin your hair over to one side like Shelly Gruwell. Her style keeps the attractive look of long hair while still allowing full view of the trapezius muscles. A woman's crowning glory—her hair—is an asset that shouldn't be ignored.

All these suggestions have a central theme: contest preparation includes making sure every detail about your appearance is planned and perfected. Don't waste all that dieting and training through a presentation that's anything less than your best!

Surviving a Contest Diet

by Claudia Cornwell Wilbourn

I could hardly believe how far women's bodybuilding had come. "Aren't they fabulous?" Joe Weider said as we watched the 1981 American Women's Bodybuilding Championship in Las Vegas. "Would you ever have thought that women could be so muscular and yet look so beautiful and feminine?"

I had to agree. The women did look great. But looking closer, seeing the stress and fatigue on their faces as they came offstage and let down their guard, I knew how high the cost of competing must have been.

I knew because I had gone through it myself. The year before I had competed for the American title. I was one of those who felt drawn, tired, depleted of energy, counting the hours until I could relax and return to a healthier, more natural way of life.

The stress of the competition itself had something to do with this. Competition on this level—whether in bodybuilding or any other sport—is psychologically arduous. The newspapers were calling me "the favorite," people with microphones and cameras were continually following me around, which put enormous pressure on me to do well in the competition.

The stress of training intensely for eight months without a break also was taking its toll. First came the Atlantic City competition, in which I placed third; then the California state contest, which I was able to win. And then I prepared for the America, during which time I ate, worked and slept competition. Every night in my dreams I stood onstage, sometimes not knowing what I was supposed to do, forgetting my posing routine.

But I had been training for more than five years, so my body should have been able to handle the strain of hard workouts. And I was old enough and experienced enough that I should have been able to handle the stress and pressures of competition.

None of these factors, by themselves, should have affected me so severely. However, there was a factor I had underestimated in planning my strategy—the enormously debilitating effect of a serious bodybuilding diet.

Dieting for bodybuilding is hard enough on men. For women, it can be disastrous. The human female naturally carries a great deal more fat than does the male. Her biochemical makeup, with its higher levels of estrogen and other hormones, makes getting extremely lean very difficult. (It's even more difficult for women taking estrogen-based oral contraceptives.) If you don't know the right way to lower your bodyfat level, if you subject your body to unnecessary abuse, the dieting process can be dangerous as well as uncomfortable.

For me, diet time was often panic time. Would I be able to lose enough subcutaneous fat to come in cut up? Could I somehow hasten the process? During the long year of training, that endless year, I became so anxious that I tried a shortcut—prescription amphetamines. Speed. My doctor gave me the strongest pills available. They were incredibly potent, with half a capsule affecting me for more than 12 hours.

The pills soon became a habit. I raced through my workouts like a madwoman. People noticed a deterioration in my personality. I was constantly nervous and excited, a high-tension wire, crackling hot and ready to snap. Midnight would come, and I would lie in bed, unable to sleep, my heart pounding audibly.

To monitor my progress, I took body composition tests. And I was shocked to find that my diet was costing me more muscle than fat! I was losing the muscle tissue that had taken years of sweat and strain to build and develop.

Obviously, I was doing something wrong. There must be something more to dieting than starvation and dangerous drugs. I stopped taking the amphetamines (and stopped seeing that doctor). I still had time to get in shape for the America, so I decided to learn how to become lean using a more healthy combination of good nutrition and exercise.

One problem was that I had no role models. The only other women with this problem were my fellow competitors—and most of them knew less about diet than I did. And now, almost two years later, I am sometimes appalled at how little the women have learned about eliminating bodyfat without burning up their muscle tissue and endangering their health.

No matter what anyone says, you have to diet to be a good bodybuilder—male or female. When a bodybuilder flexes, something has to happen, or else the judges have nothing on which to base their decision. Even with insufficient dieting you may achieve some definition and muscle separation, which may look great backstage. But once you get onstage under those lights—especially television lights—if you aren't cut to ribbons, the detail of your muscle development is totally wiped out and you might as well not have bothered dieting at all.

Women bodybuilders don't need to achieve the extremely low bodyfat level of their male counterparts, but they must make comparable percentage reductions. An average woman has 22–24% bodyfat level, but a female bodybuilder must drop to a 7–11% level for competitive success. By comparison, the average man has 15% bodyfat, while the successful male bodybuilder has 3–5%.

Dieting is necessary to achieve these low bodyfat levels, but it's an extreme process that must be approached with caution. You have to cut down on your calorie intake, but you can't starve yourself. Otherwise, you rob yourself of the energy you need to train and you cause your body to metabolize muscle tissue.

Drastic reduction methods are health hazards. For example, "bulemia," a practice first recorded by the ancient Romans, consists of gorging, then vomiting and purging to control weight. Habitual self-induced vomiting, which is epidemic among young college women, has been used by both male and female bodybuilders. Diuretics and laxatives have been used to excess, causing potassium depletion, changes in bowel habits, dehydration, muscle weakness, possible heart arrhythmia, cardiac arrest and death.

Frequently, bodybuilders try extreme regimens like the zero-carb diet. Readers of *Muscle & Fitness* no doubt know that this leads to all sorts of complications, one of which is the body's absolute need to break down and metabolize muscle tissue.

I had to learn all of this the hard way. By trial and error, I found that the only way to cut up successfully, especially for a woman, involves a balanced and sensible approach to diet and exercise. The program I ultimately arrived at includes these steps:

Plan Ahead—There are no shortcuts to fat loss. A quick weight loss will probably be as much water and muscle tissue as fat. To protect your muscle mass, don't expect more than a two-pound fat loss per week. This means you will probably have to diet 6–12 weeks to get into contest condition.

Establish a Sensible Diet—Moderate changes in your diet can have greater results than more drastic approaches. Cut back on fats and oils—they contain too many calories. Eat a balanced diet consisting of:

    50–70% carbohydrates
    22–30% protein

The carbohydrates should be complex carbs, such as vegetables and potatoes, and simple carbs, such as fruit. Foods like fish and chicken contain good protein and relatively little fat. Unprocessed foods are better than processed foods. Whole-grain bread and rice are better than white bread and processed rice.

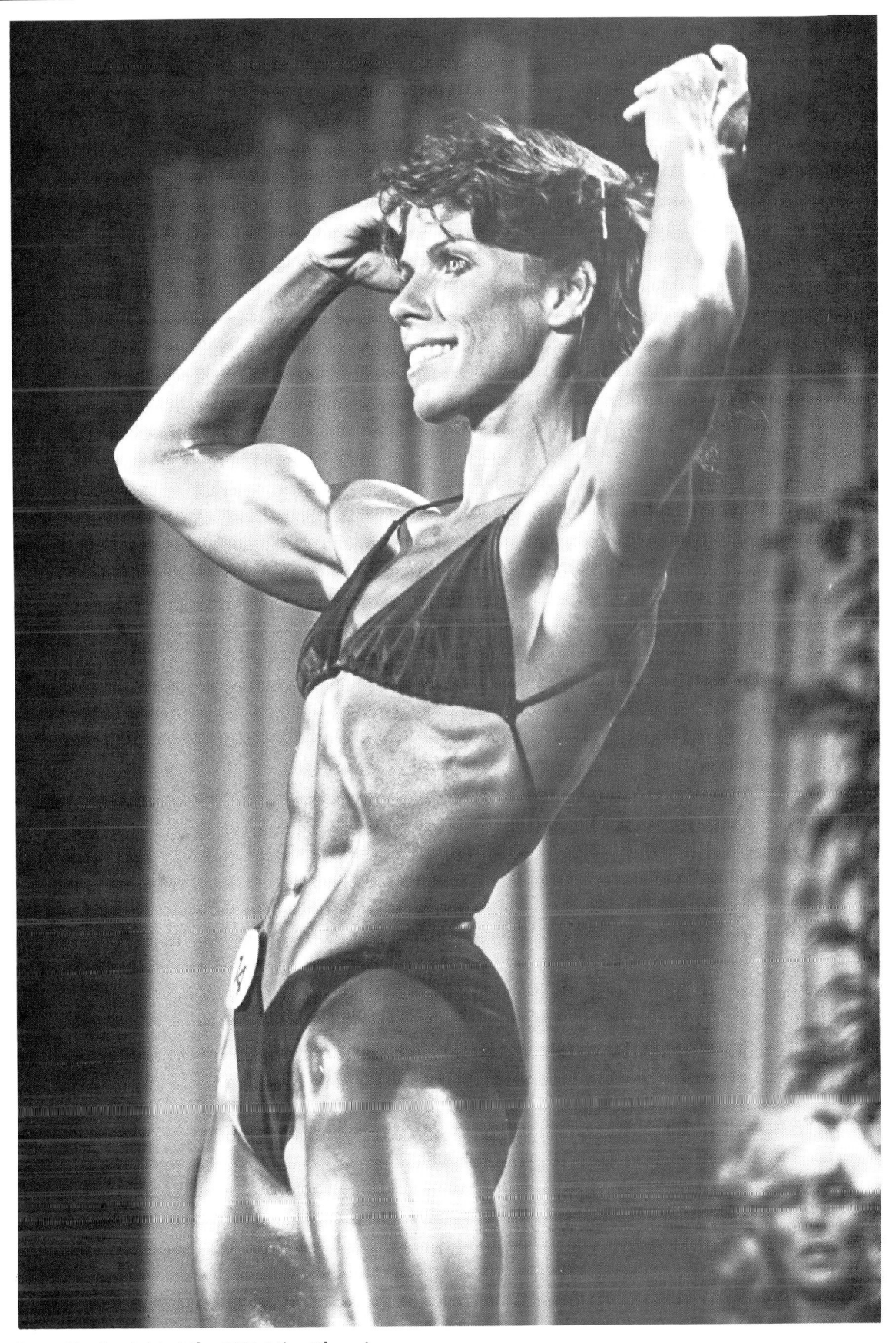

Lynn Conkwright at the 1981 Miss Olympia.

Above all, remember the difference between reducing calories and starving yourself. Eating small meals four to six times a day is much more preferable than going without food for long periods.

Increase Aerobic Exercise—Moderate, rhythmic exercise, in addition to your workouts in the gym, helps you to get lean by burning up excess calories. Research has shown that low-intensity exercise over a period of time (bicycle riding, jogging, aerobics classes) actually uses fat (as a direct source of fuel) in much higher proportions than carbohydrates.

Keep Training Intensely—Don't switch to light weights and super-high reps near a contest. Your body built muscle in response to training with heavy resistance, and it takes heavy resistance to maintain that muscle. Use diet and aerobic exercise to get rid of fat and hard workouts to build and maintain your muscles.

Get Enough Sleep—Going without rest produces symptoms much like those associated with amphetamine use. If you burn up too much nervous energy during the day, you are likely to exhaust your glucose stores. This can keep you from increasing your muscle mass, so be certain to get enough sleep. In addition, rest or meditate during the day. Staying calm and collected can help to counteract the stress of the precompetition period.

Take Body Composition Tests—Monitoring your progress with hydrostatic weighing will tell you whether you are gaining muscle and losing fat. Weighing yourself on a scale doesn't tell you whether weight changes involve muscle, fat or water.

Practice Posing—Practice your posing routine at least 15–30 minutes daily. Learn to flex and control every single muscle in your body. This will not only help your presentation immensely once you get onstage, but will also help to harden, develop and define the muscles involved.

Peaking for a contest is no magic trick, but the result of a thorough yet moderate plan followed over a sufficient period of time. I had to learn this the hard way—from my mistakes. I had no choice, because the knowledge I needed simply wasn't available. There was nobody there to teach me.

Women who are competing today have no such excuse. The knowledge is there. You must learn the fundamentals of both training and diet. You can't expect to become a top champion overnight. So don't rely on shortcuts. And once you've hung in there long enough to become knowledgeable and experienced, learn to listen to and trust your own body. Women champions, too, depend on the Weider Instinctive Principle.

You can't be blamed for making mistakes. The only fault lies in failing to learn from them.

Diuretics:
Looking Ripped Could Do You In!

by Dr. Lynne Pirie, D.O.

Early last spring Heinz Sallmayer, the 1980 IFBB Lightweight Mr. Universe, died of a heart attack while preparing for a professional competition. In his early 30s and a lifetime athlete, Sallmayer was hardly a candidate for a heart attack. An autopsy revealed a minor congenital heart malformation. But the cause of death was excessive use of diuretics, which led to heart arrhythmia (irregular heartbeat) and the heart attack.

A few weeks later Andreas Cahling reported that an 18-year-old male Swedish bodybuilder also suffered a fatal heart seizure following a competition in Stockholm. Again, massive dehydration from using potent diuretics was pegged as the cause of death.

I've personally seen several women bodybuilders faint both backstage and onstage at high-level championships in which I've competed. After talking with them, I discovered that the common denominator was the use of diuretics.

Male bodybuilders frequently are stricken with serious and very painful muscle cramps during and after competition. And in every case this is caused by an electrolyte imbalance brought on by the use of potent prescription diuretics.

As the two cited cases show, the process of dehydration before a bodybuilding competition, especially by using potent diuretics, is extremely dangerous. I warn you to beware of attempting to cut up in this manner. There are much safer and healthier methods that you can use to achieve peak muscularity onstage for your next competition.

Talk to any competitive bodybuilder about how to maximize contest definition, and he or she will no doubt tell you about dehydration. There are a number of methods used to maximize water loss from the body's tissues. Many of them are not without immediate side effects; some carry the potential for long-term kidney damage; a few are life-threatening.

Unfortunately many bodybuilders are completely in the dark about the untoward effects of body dehydration, yet they readily advise one another on how to do it. Because of this lack of knowledge, bodybuilders have been known to exercise in rubber suits, sit in saunas for prolonged periods, indiscriminately use potent diuretics, restrict salt and eliminate or severely curtail fluid intake.

A recent magazine article described a well-known bodybuilder trying to get cut up at the last minute for a major competition by sitting clad in a rubber suit in front of an oven. Such extreme approaches to dehydration are both unhealthy and unsafe.

Exercising in a hot gym, sitting in a sauna or wearing a rubber suit will knock out the normal thermostatic mechanism that controls body temperature. As a result of this tampering with the body's natural thermometer, the body's core temperature can be elevated six to eight degrees. The function of the thermoregulation system is impaired, making heat stroke and circulatory collapse a possibility. If this occurs, the major organ systems of the body will not receive an adequate blood supply and may be damaged.

Individuals who have been using diuretics, thyroid hormones, amphetamines, antihistamines, tricyclic antidepressives and other drugs are even more prone to developing heat stroke when the core temperature is elevated through some of the commonly used bodybuilding dehydration techniques. In addition to irreversible organ damage, you can also die from heat stroke or circulatory collapse.

Abusing diuretics—especially the more potent ones such as Lasix—can bring on several biochemical and physiological health problems. Electrolyte imbalance is a frequently occurring side effect, especially in bodybuilders who are also adhering to severely restricted precontest diets. The loss of the electrolyte potassium from the system can precipitate arrhythmia.

Electrolyte profiles of athletes in other sports who have abused potent diuretics to make weight for competition show seriously low amounts of sodium, potassium, calcium and chloride in the blood. The acidity of the blood has also been decreased, resulting in alkalosis, a condition of increased alkalinity of the blood and tissues.

These imbalances are reflected in fatigue, thirst, irritability, muscular cramping, gastrointestinal upsets and irregular heartbeat—all of which the average bodybuilder dismisses as part of the price he or she has to pay to achieve peak muscularity. This attitude seems very inappropriate for someone who desires the appearance of a healthy bodybuilder, however.

Oddly enough, bodybuilders tend to ignore the fact that dehydration diminishes the size of their muscles, even though muscle mass is a highly prized quality in competition. Muscles are mostly water, and depletion of water from the body's tissues decreases the volume of each muscle. Again, this seems very inappropriate for serious bodybuilders.

Diuretics can quickly deplete the circulation blood volume to such a low level that there will be no significant blood supply to the kidneys. Tests on dehydrated athletes have demonstrated impaired renal function that could possibly be permanent. Kidneys do not regenerate like the skin and hair. This decreased blood volume is a direct result of dehydration and/or the use of potent diuretics, which significantly reduce the kidneys' ability to reabsorb salt.

Diuretic use results in lower water volume in all the body's tissues, which can also cause a dizzy feeling when you get up quickly from a seated or lying position. There simply isn't enough blood in the vascular system to fully oxygenate the brain when a rapid change of body position occurs, and this is why some athletes faint at a competition.

All the foregoing effects are even more pronounced when you also restrict your salt and fluid intake. If blood volume is decreased sufficiently, circulatory collapse is again a possibility, as it is in the case of the heat stroke discussed earlier. But now there is also the chance of the formation of a lethal blood clot that can become lodged in an artery between the heart and lungs, or in the circulatory system to the brain, which would result in a stroke.

Each of the dehydration rituals described—the use of heat, rubber suits and/or potent diuretics by naive individuals—is absolutely contraindicated. This is no exaggeration. Only a physician should prescribe diuretics, and when he or she does so such biological parameters as thermoregulation, electrolyte balance and kidney function should be closely monitored.

Lasix is the most commonly used diuretic and a very potent one. Taken orally it begins to act within an hour, and peak effect is experienced within two hours. The effects of Lasix taken orally will last six to eight hours.

Injected intravenously, Lasix begins to act within five minutes, and peak effect is within an hour. Usually the effect of injected Lasix lasts about two hours.

Lasix is *not* indicated for use by people getting ready for a bodybuilding contest. The harmful effects of this diuretic are just too great to warrant its use in athletics. If a person is allergic to sulfa drugs, for example, he or she may also have an allergic reaction to Lasix. If a person is taking aspirin in addition to Lasix, there is a great risk of going into salicylate toxicity. And Lasix can increase the glucose level of the blood, which can be particularly hazardous for an undiagnosed diabetic.

Lasix has been shown to cause deformities in an unborn fetus, so it's not indicated for use by pregnant women or even by women of childbearing age, unless it's for a medical emergency. You can have a hearing loss, both reversible and irreversible, on Lasix. And, the drug can precipitate an attack of gout if a patient is prone to that disease.

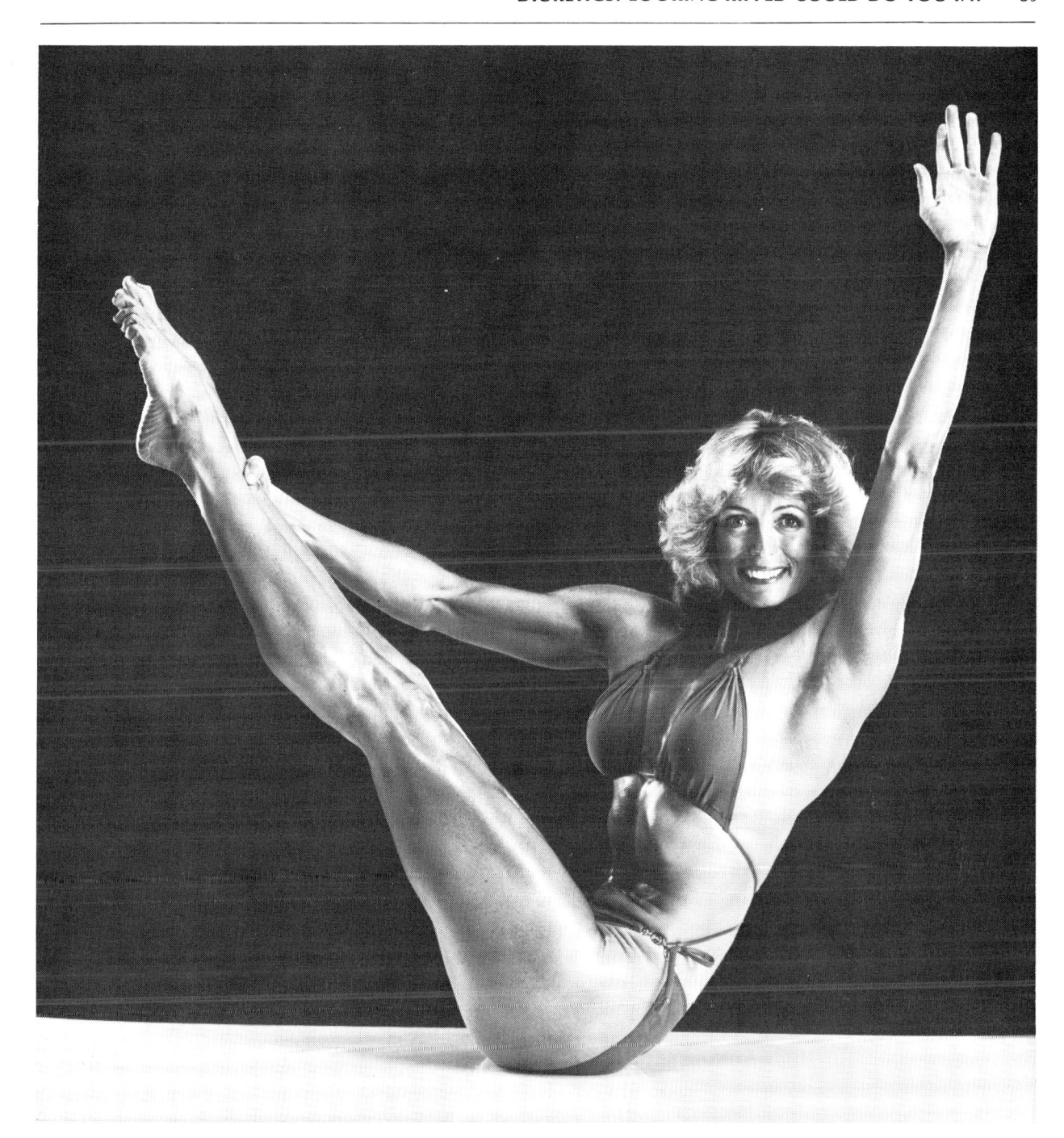

With Lasix and other harsh chemical diuretics, you can lose many of the electrolytes your body needs for proper function. You can lose calcium in the urine and get very bad muscle cramps as a result. And you can lose sodium and potassium. Without enough potassium, you can develop arrhythmia and thereby risk heart seizure. Some bodybuilders think they can counteract this by taking supplemental potassium, but they're just doing it by the seat of their pants without knowing how much they should take.

Overall, taking Lasix and other potent prescription diuretics is putting yourself in great risk. So, what can you do to achieve maximum muscularity onstage at a competition without chancing the untoward effects of diuretic use and other methods of dehydration? Well, I do have an answer to that question, and there is a bonus that goes with it—you will look, feel and act much healthier onstage if you follow my recommendations.

Mainly, you must continue on a well-balanced, low-calorie diet for long enough to deplete subcutaneous bodyfat naturally. As Joe Weider says, most bodybuilders take diuretics because they're not disciplined enough to diet for a long period, or they don't start a diet soon enough and end up too fat close to a contest.

There's a way to control the use of diuretics by bodybuilders too lazy to diet, and that is to medically test kidney function and urine concentration to determine if someone has been taking diuretics. But sometimes I wonder how strict we should be in evaluating athletes, even if we do so for their own good.

It would be far better for you as a bodybuilder to resolve to protect your precious health by avoiding diuretics and other methods of dehydration by following a well-balanced, low-calorie diet long enough to become truly cut up. This is the method used by Boyer Coe. Boyer has never used a diuretic, yet he is incredibly cut for important competitions.

Depending on how fat you've allowed yourself to get in the off-season, you should begin to diet at least three months before your competition. This will allow you to slowly bring your bodyfat down, and without having to go on too strict a diet. You can also go on a low-sodium diet (but no less than two grams of salt intake per day), which involves avoiding high-sodium foods and not using additional salt.

A woman athlete who's retaining water due to her menstrual cycle can safely use a mild herbal diuretic for two or three days before competing. Of the prescription diuretics, the only one I'd feel safe in prescribing is Dyazide, with which you don't excrete potassium. All you lose is salt and water. I recommend taking no more than one or two of these tablets per day for one or two days before a contest, depending on how bloated a woman happens to be.

Overall, if you do feel that you need to take a diuretic, use only a mild herbal diuretic for two or three days. Avoid overheating your body by wearing vapor barriers, training in a hot gym or spending inordinate amounts of time in a sauna. The use of potent diuretics and other common methods of dehydration by bodybuilders preparing for a contest is very dangerous.

In sum, avoid diuretics. Your health comes first, and bodybuilding should be a health-promoting sport. Let's keep it that way!

Female Factors in Bodybuilding

by Dr. Lynne Pirie, D.O.

As a physician and a competitive bodybuilder, I'm quite interested in a variety of specifically female concerns related to bodybuilding and weight training.

BIRTH CONTROL

Many women take birth-control pills. However, the estrogen and progesterone content of these pills can cause significant fluid retention, especially near the end of the cycle. A woman bodybuilder doesn't know if the extra weight is bodyfat or retained water, and she has great difficulty timing her conditioning peak under such circumstances.

Few women understand that progesterone has a protein catabolic effect. In other words, it breaks down muscle tissue, the exact opposite of what a bodybuilder wants. No serious woman bodybuilder should use oral contraceptives containing progesterone.

Other conditions, often evident in a woman's medical history, also preclude the use of birth-control pills. One is the possibility of blood clotting. If you are dehydrating—and many women bodybuilders use a diuretic to bring out the maximum degree of muscular definition—you increase thromboembolic potential (your body's potential to form blood clots).

Blood clots are likely to be very small, but they can also be large. Small clots can damage various organs, such as the spleen, liver, kidneys or any organ through which blood flows. Larger clots can cause strokes by shutting off blood to the brain. If a woman is taking *both* birth-control pills and anabolic steroids, she is risking enormous damage. I don't know of research specifically aimed at this problem, but I can tell you that this combination throws the whole endocrine system out of balance. You're changing your entire hormonal environment. If you have a dormant tumor and it responds to the new environment, it will grow with disastrous consequences. You're also destroying your entire neural-hormonal axis, which can affect every organ system in your body. In short, steroids are much more dangerous for a woman who's taking birth-control pills than for one who isn't.

What birth-control method should a sexually active woman bodybuilder use? The IUD (intrauterine device) was once considered quite safe, but we know now that an IUD always poses a danger of perforation of the uterus, or of the body expelling the device. An IUD is made of metal or plastic and is foreign to the human body, so the uterus may try to reject it.

Sometimes IUDs have actually gone through the wall of the uterus, and if the perforation is serious enough, a hysterectomy may be necessary. IUDs are also suspected of contributing to inflammations that can cause infertility. If a woman has never had children, that's a very high price to pay.

I recommend the use of a diaphragm. It's a minor inconvenience at times, but takes only a couple of minutes to insert. Correctly used, a diaphragm is an effective birth-control device. And, in a health sense, it is safe to use one.

MENSTRUATION

Can exercise and diet affect a woman's menstrual function? Yes! to a certain degree they can promote menstruation and ease discomfort, but at extreme levels they can disrupt the process.

There appears to be an optimal level of exercise that assists menstruation and relieves menstrual complications, but still doesn't interfere with menstrual function. The menstrual cramps younger women often have can definitely be eased by exercise, but excessive exercise can affect the menstrual cycle.

Certain anti-inflammatory foodstuffs, such as wine and the amino acid tryptophane, can relieve menstrual cramping slightly. Overall, however, exercise does a better job of relieving cramps.

Bodybuilding, track, gymnastics and other sports that require a low bodyweight and involve a high degree of stress can cause amenorrhea, or a cessation of menses. This is probably due to a very quick weight loss and/or general stress.

Delayed menses are relatively common among girls who are serious dancers, gymnasts, runners, or who participate in other strenuous sports and must maintain a low degree of bodyfat. A certain height-weight ratio apparently must be achieved before such a young woman will menstruate.

Amenorrhea

There has been considerable speculation on whether or not an amenorrheic woman ovulates, but there is no scientific evidence to support either stand. Therefore, it would be foolish to assume that amenorrhea is an effective birth-control system. Without relying on other forms of birth control, you could become pregnant.

All the investigation I've done on amenorrhea indicates it isn't dangerous. The menses simply seem to resume as soon as a woman's bodyweight goes back up.

Unfortunately, many gynecologists aren't experienced in treating amenorrhea, and they immediately prescribe hormonal therapy to induce menses. Such a procedure is both expensive and unnecessary. To resume your menses, simply gain bodyweight and perhaps reduce your level of physical activity.

Menopause

There has been little research on the relationship between exercise and menopause, and none on the relationship between bodybuilding and menopause. I can, however, give you an informed opinion.

Menopause is a time of general deterioration of the body as a consequence of the natural aging process. Bodybuilding works in the opposite direction: it promotes tissue growth rather than atrophy. Thus, regular bodybuilding and weight training will probably help minimize the negative effects of menopause.

PREGNANCY

When a woman bodybuilder embarks on a new type of "bodybuilding"—pregnancy, that is—should she continue her weight training? If she's been training regularly prior to pregnancy, she can profitably continue to work out. It's not a good idea, however, for an out-of-shape woman to commence hard training after she discovers she's pregnant. A pregnant woman shouldn't do anything that she's not used to physically. It's important to avoid overtraining, which can cause anoxia (a deficit of oxygen) to the fetus.

Many woman athletes have continued to train fairly vigorously up to and through the seventh and eighth months of their pregnancies. The better a woman's musculature, the better control she can have over her own delivery. This also takes into consideration such athletic-related abilities as self-control, self-discipline and the ability to control pain. A woman who's in very good physical condition can push down harder and deliver more quickly. There's a lot of pain associated with childbirth, and a woman who is used to training in pain can handle it better.

Nutritionally, a woman bodybuilder should adjust her diet as any other pregnant woman would, and that includes increasing her intake of folic acid and other vitamins. A pregnant woman bodybuilder should not be dieting—or training—for a contest. This should be quite obvious, but it must be said nonetheless, considering the

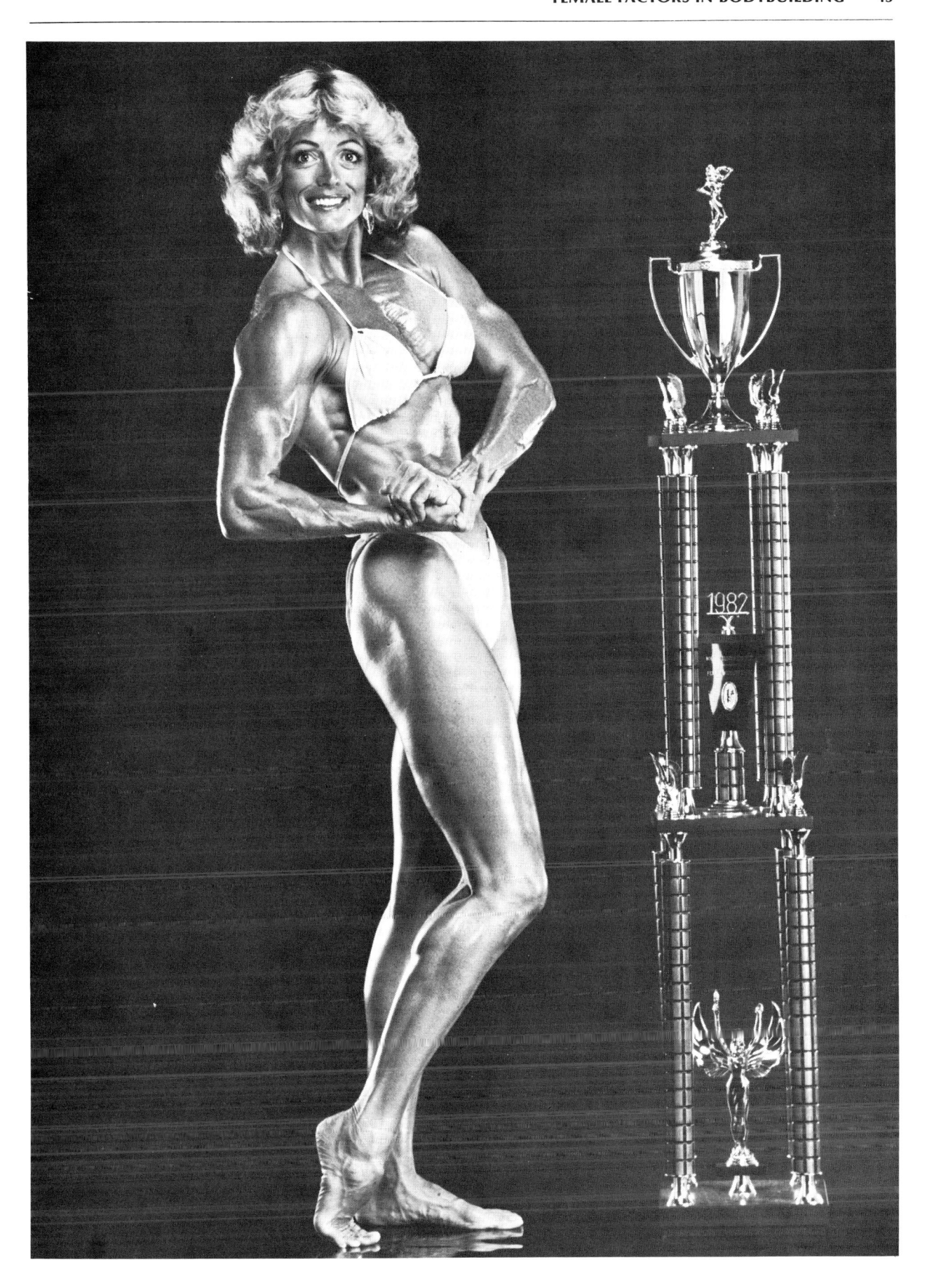

FEMALE FACTORS IN BODYBUILDING 43

competitive nature and enthusiasm of most bodybuilders.

Childbirth

After giving birth, all women are concerned with regaining their pre-pregnancy appearance and physical condition. It will be easy for a bodybuilder to accomplish this, because any woman who remained in excellent physical condition during her pregnancy will have a full and rapid recovery following childbirth. Numerous champion women bodybuilders have regained such superb condition after pregnancy that they've been consistent winners in bodybuilding competition.

ANOREXIA NERVOSA

Anorexia nervosa, a mental-physical disease that affects primarily women (and more women from the upper middle class than from any other socioeconomic group), has gained considerable publicity in recent years. It is characterized by prolonged fasting or subsistence on a bare minimum of calories, as well as by frequent endurance-type exercise, all aimed at making an anorexic "fashionably thin." As the disorder becomes progressively more serious, it can be life-threatening.

While I personally know of no anorexic women bodybuilders, the requirements of the sport (strict dieting and copious exercise) can lead to anorexia nervosa. If a woman becomes anorexic, it's not something that should be handled by a friend in the gym, or even by a family physician. In my opinion, anorexia nervosa is a psychiatric emergency that should be treated only by a psychiatrist specifically experienced with handling the disorder. In many cases an anorexic should actually be hospitalized.

Anorexia nervosa is often difficult for a family member to identify because anorexics become very devious about disguising their symptoms. They'll even begin to pad their clothing to hide the fact that they're losing so much weight.

Bulemia is a related disease that also should be treated psychiatrically. Bulemics will gorge themselves with food and then cause the food to be regurgitated by sticking a finger down the throat. As with anorexia nervosa, this is a potentially serious disorder that could be related to women in competitive bodybuilding, as well as in a variety of other sports.

"We're Training Partners and Proud of It!"

by Claudia Cornwell Wilbourn

"Why I Train with Men" was an article I wrote for *Muscle & Fitness* in 1979. It was the first opportunity I had to work with Joe Weider, and was I thrilled! A few women bodybuilders such as Lisa Lyon, Stacey Bentley and myself had captured the attention of the media. Joe Weider was the first magazine publisher in the bodybuilding/fitness field to allow us to express our viewpoints—our motivations, struggles and goals in the nascent sport of female bodybuilding.

In that article, I explained why I trained with men and found their assistance invaluable. After years of being the only woman in bodybuilding gyms, I was proud that men accepted me. That seemed to vindicate my dedication and seriousness. The sport was dominated by men—they had the expertise in training, posing and conducting seminars. So it seemed natural that women should turn to men as mentors.

Women's bodybuilding has progressed faster than any of us could have imagined, however. Part of the sport's growth is reflected in patterns of behavior in bodybuilding gyms around the world: Women are no longer rarities in a gym. Now a new trend is evident—women training with women. This is not a reference to the health spa social hour that passes for a workout. Serious female athletes are training with one another and benefiting from the partnership.

Miss Olympia winner Rachel McLish often trains with AFWB President Susan Fry. Kay Baxter, a top professional bodybuilder, values her female training partners, as do many other prominent women athletes. I too have come a long way from my misogynist perspective back in '79. Workouts with my female partner are some of the most intense and satisfying I have ever experienced. This says something considering that I have had the privilege of training with such men as Samir Bannout, Pete Grymkowski, Bill Grant, Andreas Cahling and Casey Viator.

Women training together is a trend both significant and timely. Women are now viewing other women less as adversaries and more as sisters in need of support. The female sport puts less emphasis on getting the edge on other women, or attempting to diminish their development. Instead we focus on becoming the most we can be with the help of other women.

The proliferation of women's networks—groups of women with common interests gathering together—has influenced women's awareness of one another in general. These groups allow professional or nonprofessional women to share their concerns and gain an insight into their field. Now female bodybuilders have created their own network. This is important because for many bodybuilding is a world of discovery. Women can learn to *do*

45

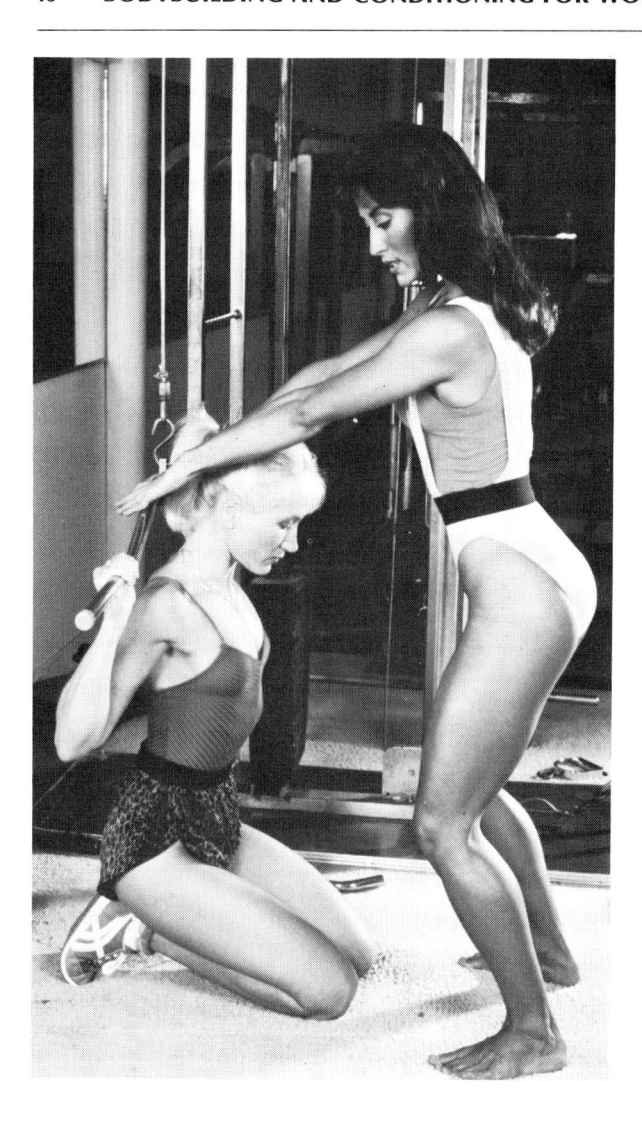

rather than *be*, to discover their bodies through an exploration of endurance, strength and muscle function.

It is appropriate for bodybuilding women to share with one another, because men have not experienced the same restrictions to development: Men have traditionally been encouraged to find themselves through athletics, the military and high-risk occupations. In *Machisma: Women and Daring*, Grace Lichtenstein emphasizes that boys are taught to seek their own limits and uncover their own strengths in the company of other males. Consequently, men are rarely estranged from their bodies as are women.

It is not uncommon for women to attribute all positive influences to maleness. There is a tendency to see men as Merlins, to think that they hold the magic key to power and success. Girls have been culturally encouraged to seek a strong male and derive her worth, identity and life direction from him. We have felt honored to participate in men's games and activities because of our respect for the strong assertive male image.

Male bodybuilders *have* been very helpful to women by teaching us training techniques, posing fundamentals, etc. Female bodybuilding would not be where it is today if men in the sport had not led the way. Nonetheless, the sport needs female role models, with compassion for their sisters, women who take risks and help redefine the feminine experience.

Kay Baxter sees a change in the way women regard one another. She recently told me:

"There's a growing camaraderie. I believe what we've been taught is a myth—that women cannot trust other women. We *can* trust one another. There's a sisterhood out there! It's a kind of enlightened new perspective nowhere more evident than in gyms and AFWB contests. I meet with the women, and there's no nit-picking, no back stabbing.

"I used to feel very competitive with other women. I mistrusted them. It started in high school when I was trying out for cheerleading, when I was in competition with the other girls. But all those competitive feelings changed when I worked in an all-woman health club in Toronto. There was such a feeling of unity and sistership because we were all working together to better ourselves. From then on, I've preferred women as training partners. I've successfully worked out with many women, including Stacey Bentley, Andrena Hawkins and Pillow, who really helped me as I was preparing for the 1981 World Championships.

"Now I have the perfect training partner—Shannon Stember. She has a completely different body type from mine, a classic female physique with a small waist and great shape! Though she has never competed, she is as strong as I am. Every morning we train for about three hours at her boyfriend's place—Gamboa's Gym in Venice, California. We're constantly changing, revising, attacking each bodypart from a different angle. And I've never put on so much muscle in my life!"

Kay gave me three reasons why it can be preferable for women to train together:

"First, when you work out with a woman there is nothing sexual involved. You pay closer attention to the training, because you aren't distracted by a sexual attraction to your partner. And you don't worry about being too sweaty or grubby.

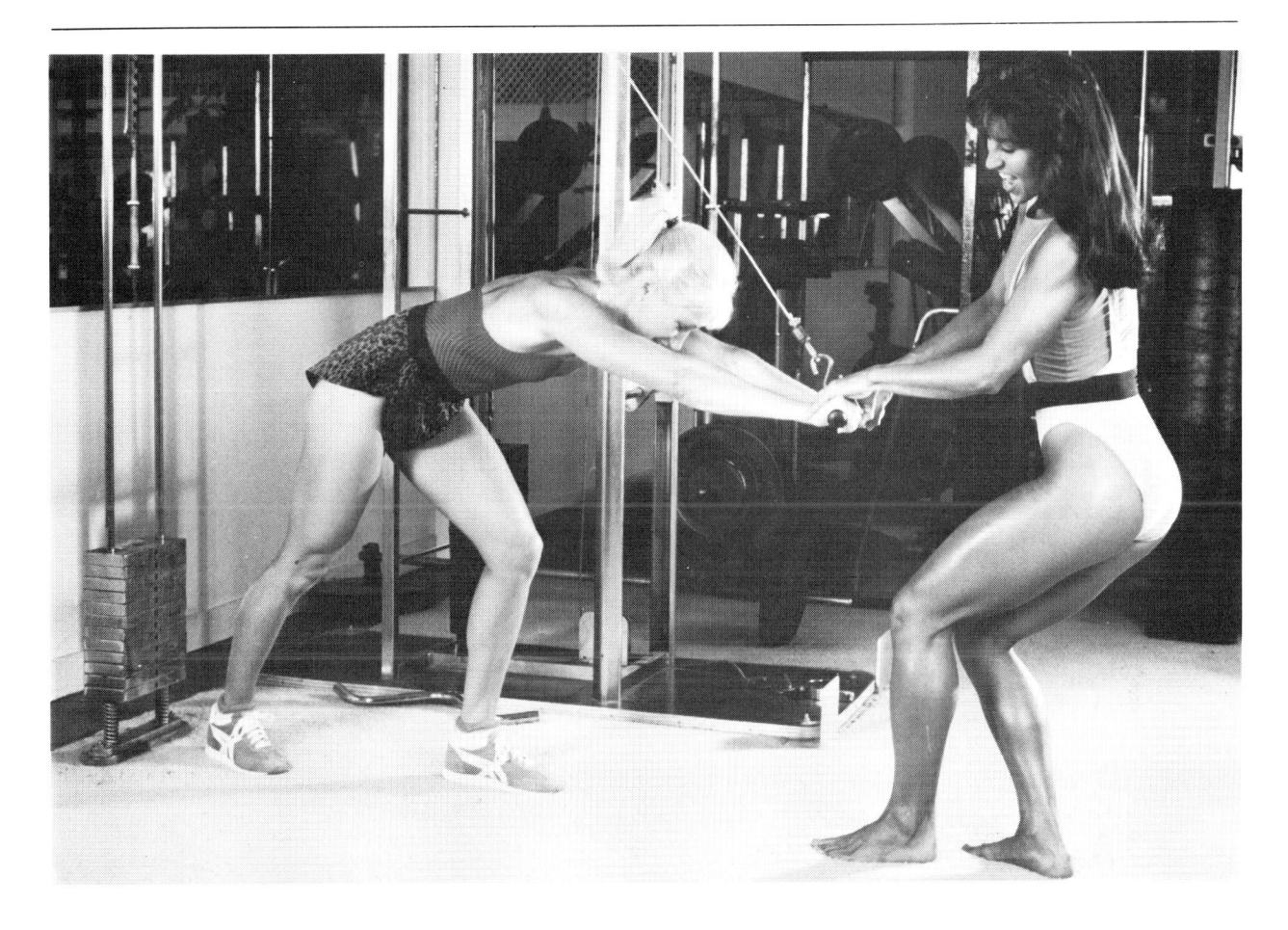

"Secondly, there is no shuffling back and forth with the weights. A lot of energy and time is saved because we use the same weights.

"Thirdly, women are generally more reliable. They let fewer things interfere with the workout. In my experience, it's been the women that I could count on."

There are more reasons for women sharing the bodybuilding experience. Men and women are different creatures who may have different needs and desires. The male "do or die" approach to athletics might not appeal to all women, since most of us have not been indoctrinated with the Vince Lombardi "winning is the only thing" credo. A woman's machisma behavior in the gym may be little more than shallow imitation of men with no reflection of her values and goals.

During those early years when I trained as the only female in bodybuilding gyms, I definitely exhibited machisma. I strutted about the gym displaying my muscles, challenging the men to tests of strength and endurance. Yet, over the years as I became more comfortable and sure of myself, I began reclaiming aspects of my personality that I had denied. I learned again to feel empathy for others. The tremendous need to prove myself strong and tough has diminished. And my style of training is no longer imitative of my male friends, but rather suits my personality and my personal outlook.

For the first time in 11 years, I have a female training partner, Linda Gearing. In the gym men tease us, calling us "Chatty Cathys." Our laughter and playfulness set us apart from the other bodybuilders. We do not buy the myth that something must always be painful and lonely to be efficiently performed. An obnoxious antagonistic demeanor does not guarantee fantastic results!

When a set is performed, my partner and I are serious and intense, giving everything to the effort! We coax each other. "Think thick! Feel those muscle fibers deep inside your chest explode! Stretch deeper! Drive it up!"

Linda and I certainly don't wander about the gym during our workout to chat with the bodybuilders. But we do have the ability to shift focus—to integrate mind and body, to be aware of physical and mental responses and developments simultaneously. As our bodies grow and respond to weight training, our awareness of ourselves as women grows. We talk about our feelings, bodily changes, anxieties and perceptions in a running dialogue. A hostile taunting approach to weight training would not be suitable for us.

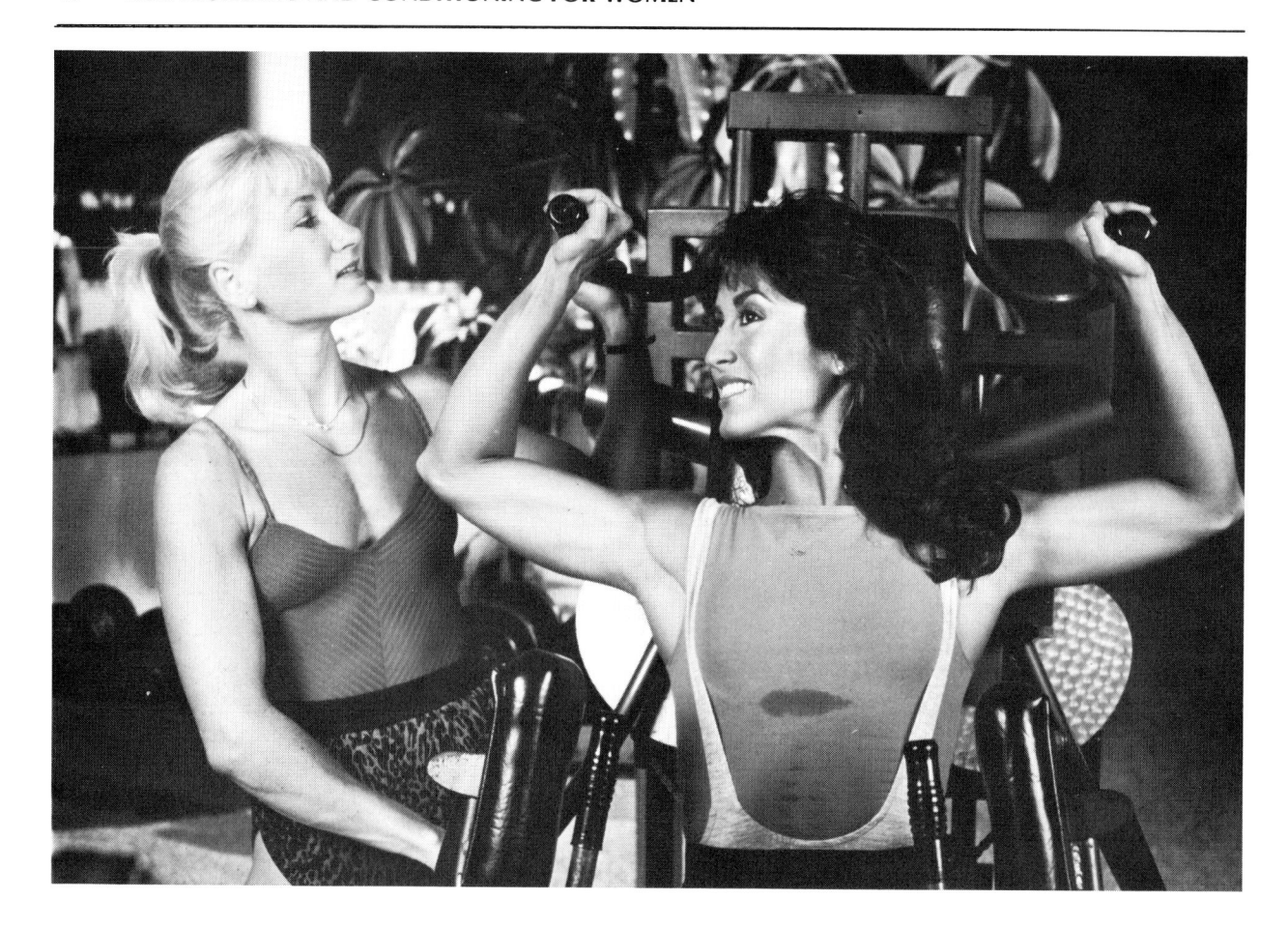

Linda has expressed her feelings concerning our partnership:

"Training with a woman is accepting the fact that you are a woman, and training your body's capacity. We're intuitive, understanding unspoken things about the other woman's body, with a caring and sensitivity a man doesn't have.

"Not only am I building my body but I'm building my mind—experiencing life fully as a woman. For me training takes on a different meaning. To be able to discuss my growth, to verbalize how I feel is like building from the inside out.

"The conversation shared between us in the gym is very special, very private. I don't have to share it with anyone else. And it's unique, it's a total development. These conversations in the gym are totally different from the ones I have with a man. There's a certain guidance that is shared: each watching out for the other, a give-and-take on equal terms.

"I have never shared so much with another woman in my whole life. I've been alienated from women. This situation is unique and exciting. While training intensely, we laugh and enjoy what we're doing."

Because bodybuilding exemplifies an important fulfillment for many women seeking personal development, it follows that there is a great desire among women bodybuilders to affiliate with other women. Seldom has there been encouragement to make connections among women, and women often feel deprived of feminine relationships.

Even at this time, female bodybuilders face condemnation and isolation as they challenge our culture's female stereotype. We need to build a supportive environment of like-minded women with whom to share, take risks, build trust. We must and *are* creating an atmosphere in which positive conflict, achievement and growth are possible. A place to test our own parameters and discover new possibilities together.

It is critical at this stage for women to train and work together, and communicate through organizations such as the AFWB. Rather than imitate a pattern of male behavior, we will invent

"WE'RE TRAINING PARTNERS AND PROUD OF IT!"

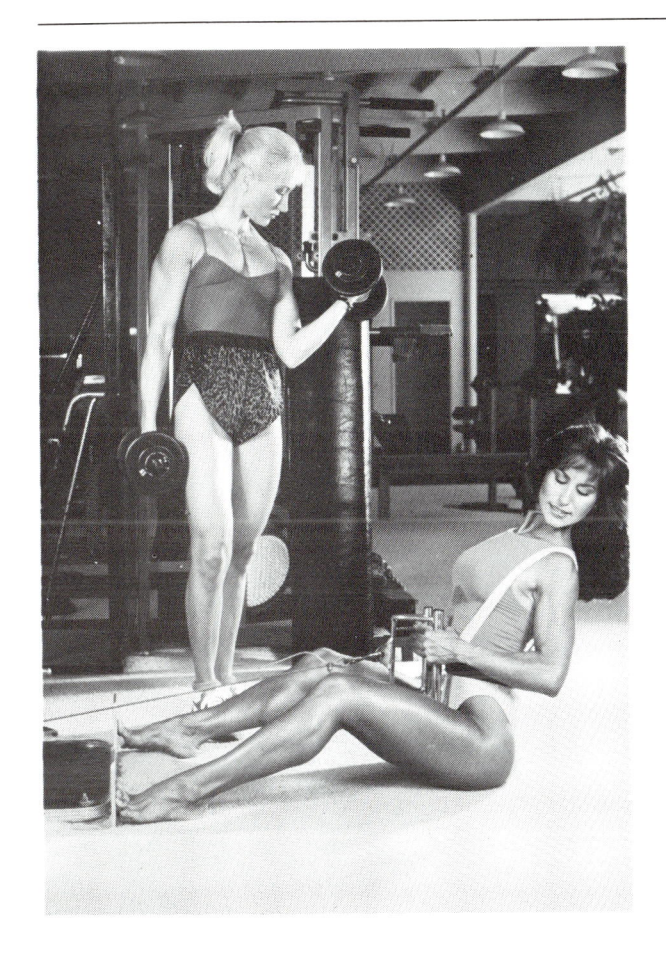

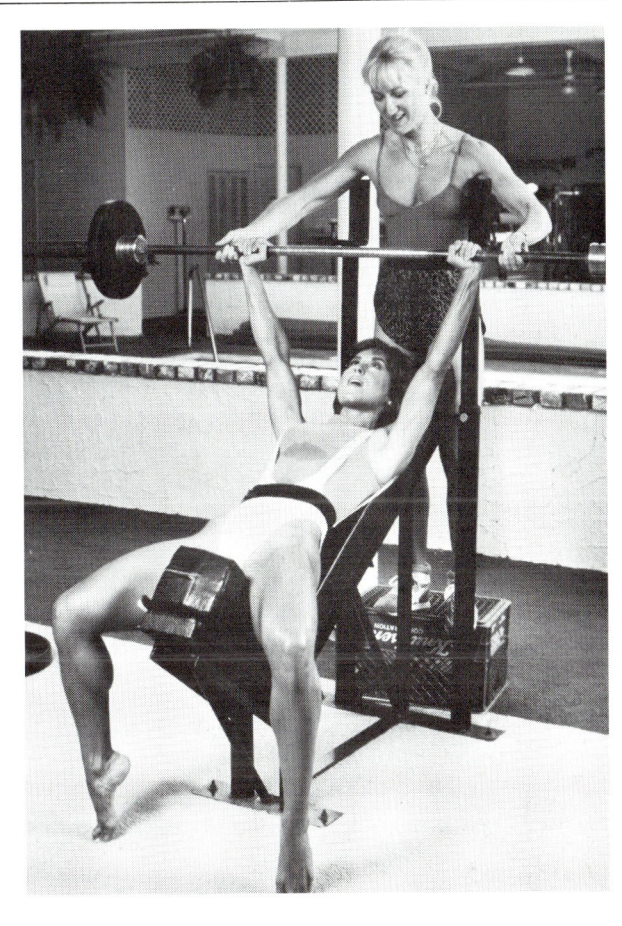

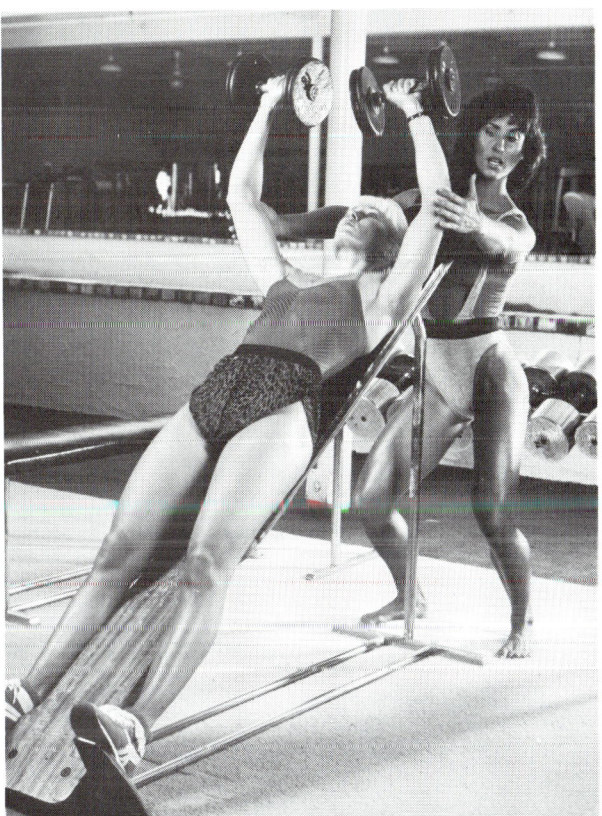

new patterns. We must establish ourselves as role models for girls entering bodybuilding by defining our experiences and our sport in our own way. Only together will we be able to challenge the American stereotype of the weak, passive woman.

Female bodybuilding has already developed its own distinct identity, with its champion athletes becoming superheroes to young men and women worldwide.

In the words of veteran bodybuilder Kay Baxter: "We haven't scratched the surface, we've dug a trench! We've come so far so fast! I believe there is distinctly a camaraderie in female bodybuilding which is not in other activities. It reminds me of my experiences as a soldier and the closeness which develops between the soldiers when they are put under stress. I have army buddies! Women for whom I have real deep feelings and respect. And I feel the same about some of the women in bodybuilding."

Susan Fry accurately sums up this sentiment and the significance of women working together: "The last frontier was not really getting into the men's weight rooms. The last frontier was facing our own sisters and realizing we're not in competition with one another, which we have always been led to believe. In bodybuilding, women discovered a whole different aspect to what it means to be a woman and relate to another woman. We have learned to let down the barriers with another woman long enough to like her, to share the benefits of our experience.

"There's a new mental awareness in the sport—not just by the women in competition but the women out there in the gyms. Weight training is like being in the Marines. The women go through something tough together and feel closer with each other than with people they see casually."

Yes, I have come a long way since 1979. Apparently many other women have had parallel experiences. Women's networks, achievements and assertive action are reflected in the sport. Female bodybuilding brings women together in a partnership of mental and physical growth. Men are a tremendous asset to our sport and can be fine trainers and workout partners, but we do have a new option—a new possibility for expansion and nurturance found only in other women.□

A Strong, Sensuous Back

by Lisa Elliott

Millions of American women suffer from lower back pains, missing countless hours of work as a result. And, ironically, almost all these back problems could be prevented through regular weight training aimed at strengthening the back muscles.

A well-developed back will add a unique sensuality to your body, and it can greatly improve your posture and athletic performance. Of course, a strong back is essential for any woman who wants to be a winner in bodybuilding competition.

In my own training I treat my back as three separate bodyparts. These are the *upper back* (primarily the trapezius muscles), the *middle back* (latissimus dorsi) and the *lower back* (erector spinae). For optimum strength, health and muscular development, all three areas must be trained in each workout.

TRAPEZIUS DEVELOPMENT

Most beginning bodybuilders and powerlifters receive sufficient trapezius stimulation from their shoulder and mid-back exercises. The Seated Pulley Row (described later) is primarily a latissimus dorsi movement, but it also strongly stresses the trapezius muscles. And all forms of Standing Presses and Lateral Raises also indirectly stimulate the trapezius muscles.

Women often ask me for exercises to correct rounded shoulders. Any trapezius movement will improve this type of postural problem, but I've found Upright Rowing to be the best exercise to improve posture. Adding one or two sets (8–10 reps per set) of this movement to your regular full-body workout will rapidly solve postural problems. Other good exercises for direct trapezius stimulation are Barbell Shoulder Shrugs, Dumbbell Shrugs and Shrugs done either on a Nautilus machine or at the Bench Press station of a Universal Gym.

Most women will never need to do more than one or two total sets of direct trapezius exercise per workout. Athletes and bodybuilders may, however, need to undertake specialized trapezius training if that area is weak or underdeveloped. Any athletic coach can identify weak muscle groups and outline a weight workout to correct them.

If your trapezius muscles are so weak that they are hindering your sports performance, try this weight routine:

Exercise	Sets	Reps
Barbell Shrugs	3	6–8
Upright Rowing	3	8–10

specialized upper back program. Here's a trapezius program that has worked well for all the women who train in the gym where I work out:

Exercise	Sets	Reps
Upright Rowing	3	8-10
Barbell Shrugs	2-3	6-8
Dumbbell Shrugs	2-3	6-8

(A couple of months of this workout would put traps on a lab skeleton.)

LATISSIMUS DORSI DEVELOPMENT

Regardless of her weight training goals, every woman should do two basic types of exercises for her latissimus dorsi muscles. Pulldown-type movements (Lat Machine Pulldowns, Chins, etc.) will develop lat width, while rowing-type exercises (Seated Pulley Rows, Barbell or Dumbbell Bent Rowing, T-Bar Rowing, etc.) promote thickness in the mid-back muscles. For optimum mid-back strength, appearance and development, both types of movements should be done in each back workout.

For greater back strength and development—as well as improved athletic ability—you can use these beginning and intermediate latissimus dorsi training routines:

Beginners (women with less than 8-10 weeks of steady training experience)

Exercise	Sets	Reps
Seated Pulley Rowing	2-3	6-8
Lat Machine Pulldown	2-3	8-10

Intermediates (women with up to six months of steady training experience)

Exercise	Sets	Reps
Dumbbell Bent Rowing	3-4	6-8
Lat Machine Pulldown	3	8-10
Seated Pulley Rowing	3	8-10

The intermediate latissimus dorsi routine just listed would develop sufficient mid-back strength for most women athletes. If you participate in a sport that places a premium on

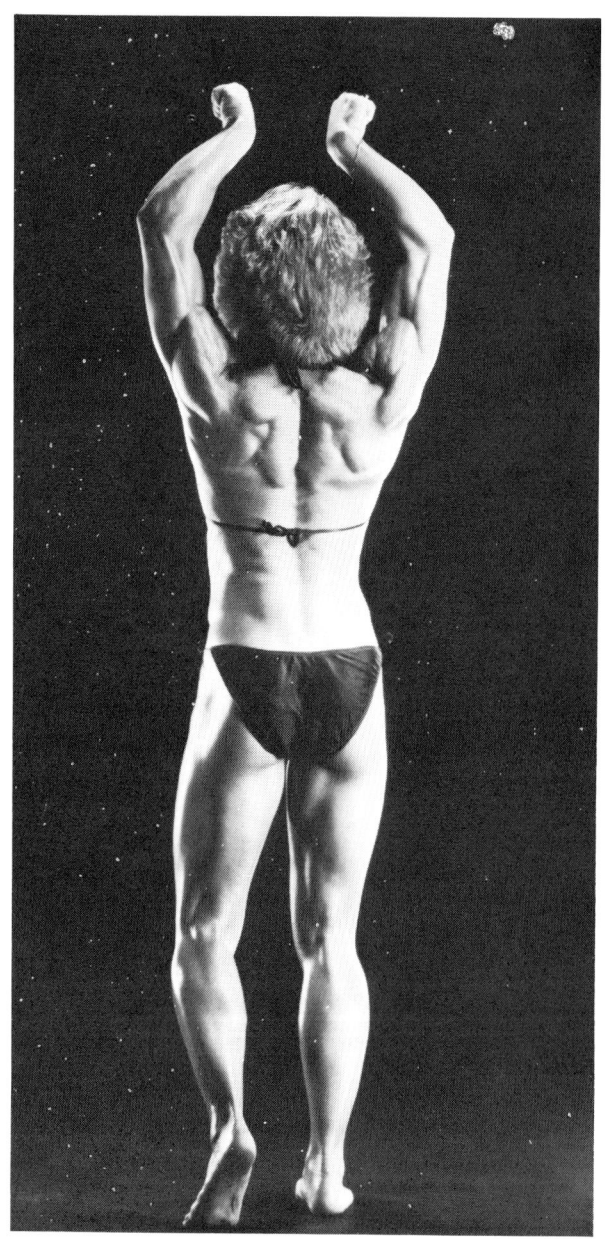

Lisa Elliott.

This routine will rapidly increase trapezius strength and will improve athletic performance in pulling-type sports such as crew.

As a competing bodybuilder I've never had to do much direct training for my traps, because my lat and deltoid training strongly stimulate this muscle. The only direct work I do for my trapezius is two or three sets (six reps per set) of some type of Shoulder Shrug. I prefer to change the type of shrugs I do from one workout to the next because this adds variety to my routines and keeps me from getting bored.

If you are a bodybuilder with lagging trapezius development, however, you must adopt a lat strength, however, you may need to do a mid-back routine like this one:

Exercise	Sets	Reps
Seated Pulley Rowing	4	6-8
Barbell Bent Rowing	3-4	6-8
Behind Neck Lat Pulldown	3-4	8-10
Front of Neck Lat Pulldown	3-4	8-10

Because my goals in competitive bodybuilding are high, my own latissimus dorsi training program is much more complex. This is how I am currently training my lats in preparation for the upcoming National Bodybuilding Championships:

Exercise	Sets	Reps
Chin Behind Neck (with up to 20 pounds of added resistance tied around my waist)	3	6
Reverse Close-Grip Lat Pulldown	3	6
Seated Pulley Rowing	3	6
T-Bar Rowing	3	6
Narrow-Grip Chins	3	6

By cutting back a set or two per exercise, any up-and-coming competitive bodybuilder or advanced weight athlete could use this same routine. Be very careful to work up slowly to my high level of training intensity, however. A less-experienced bodybuilder who tries to do my complete lat program without a breaking-in period would experience severe muscle soreness the next few days.

At the end of this article I will give a detailed description of several key back exercises. For now, you should know that the most commonly used movements for back width are Chins (behind the neck, in front of the neck, with an overgrip, with an undergrip, and with various hand spacing widths) and Lat Pulldowns (same variations). The best back thickness exercises are Bent Rows (with a barbell, two dumbbells or a single dumbbell), T-Bar Rows and Seated Pulley Rows.

ERECTOR SPINAE DEVELOPMENT

By properly strengthening your lower back, you can avoid most of the lumbar pains many women are forced to endure. I personally don't favor lower back movements that compress the spinal vertebrae. These compression movements include Deadlifts, Stiff-Legged Deadlifts and the Good Morning Exercise. Instead, I recommend Hyperextensions to improve lower back strength and development. Hyperextensions stimulate the erector spinae muscles while actually stretching the spine. You can even do Hyperextensions while experiencing mild lower back pain. A couple of sets (10-15 reps per set) of Hyperextensions will often stretch the lower back enough to relieve backaches.

A beginning weight athlete probably won't need to do any direct lower back training because the other back movements—as well as Squats for the thighs—will indirectly stimulate the lumbar muscles. At the intermediate level, any woman would profit from doing 2-3 sets (10-15 reps per set) of Hyperextensions. In fact, this is the lower back routine that I follow, since my spinal erector muscles grow in size rather easily.

If you are a bodybuilder or athlete who needs to bring up subpar lower back development and/or strength, you can try this all-out specialization routine for your erector spinae muscles:

Exercise	Sets	Reps
Hyperextension	3	10-15
Stiff-Legged Deadlifts	2-3	8-10
Good Mornings	2-3	10-12

At one point I used this routine myself, and my erector spinae muscles grew rapidly in both size and strength. After two months I could deadlift triple my bodyweight with little difficulty, which should give you an indication of how fast strength can be increased on this training program. Now I do much less lower back work.

INTEGRATED BACK WORKOUTS

In this article I have presented specialized routines for the upper, middle and lower back. This has probably been somewhat confusing for some readers, so I would like to present the following four back workouts that integrate exercises for the trapezius, latissimus dorsi and erector spinae muscles:

Beginning level (for bodybuilders, athletes and women interested in improving strength, health and appearance).

Exercise	Sets	Reps
Upright Rowing	1-2	8-10
Barbell Bent Rowing	2-3	6-8
Front of Neck Lat Pulldown	2-3	8-10

Intermediate (for the same group of women as mentioned above; minimum of 6-8 weeks of steady training experience).

Exercise	Sets	Reps
Upright Rowing	2-3	8-10
Dumbbell Shrugs	2-3	6-8
Seated Pulley Rowing	3-4	6-8
Front of Neck Lat Pulldown	3	8-10
Back of Neck Lat Pulldown	3	8-10
Hyperextensions	2-3	10-15

Lynn Conkwright at the 1981 Atlantic City Championship.

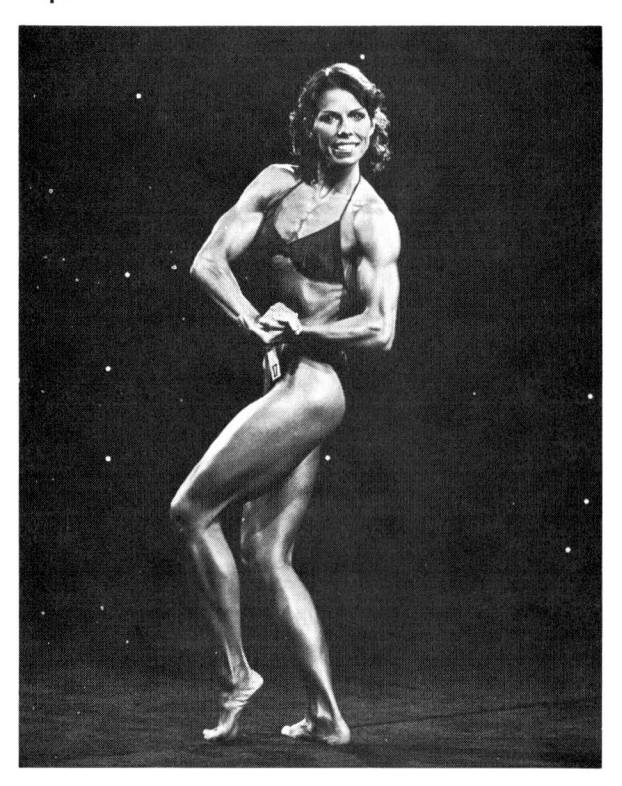

Advanced level (for bodybuilders—particularly in off-season training—and athletes with six months or more of training experience).

Exercise	Sets	Reps
Upright Rowing	3-4	8-10
Dumbbell Shrugs	3-4	6-8
Front of Neck Chins	3	6-8
Seated Pulley Rowing	3	6-8
Back of Neck Lat Pulldown	3	8-10
One-Arm Dumbbell Bent Rowing	3	8-10
Hyperextensions	3-4	10-15

Competitive level (for competing bodybuilders only).

Exercise	Sets	Reps
Upright Rowing	3	8-10
Barbell Shrugs	3	6-8
Universal Gym Shrugs	3	6-8
Back of Neck Chins	4	6-8
Barbell Bent Rowing	4	6-8
Front of Neck Lat Pulldowns	4	8-10
Seated Pulley Rowing	4	8-10
Hyperextensions	3	10-15
Stiff-Legged Deadlift	3	10-15

EXERCISE TIPS

1. Train your back two or three nonconsecutive days per week. I work my back and chest on Mondays and Thursdays. But beginners and intermediates can train their back in whole-body workouts on Mondays, Wednesdays and Fridays. A few champion women bodybuilders prefer to train their backs with their biceps and forearms twice a week, their chest, shoulders and triceps twice a week, and their legs twice a week.

2. Rest no more than 60 seconds between sets. Close to a contest I use the Weider Quality Training Principle by reducing my rest intervals between sets to as little as 20 seconds.

3. When using the Weider Supersets Training Principle, superset your back exercises with chest exercises (e.g., Chins with Bench Presses).

4. Use the Weider Overload Training Principle by constantly trying to add weight to your

movements, but not at the expense of sacrificing strict exercise form.

5. Once you get to the point where you are using substantial poundages, warm up thoroughly. A warm-up is particularly important if you do heavy Deadlifts.

6. If a part of your back—or even your entire back structure—is weak and underdeveloped, train it first in your workout (the Weider Muscle Priority Training Principle). Only at the beginning of a workout are you mentally and physically fresh enough to bomb a muscle group at peak intensity.

CONCLUSIONS

I sincerely hope that you use some of the back training advice and programs that I've outlined here. If you do, you'll quickly reach your weight training and bodybuilding goals, regardless of how high you have set them!□

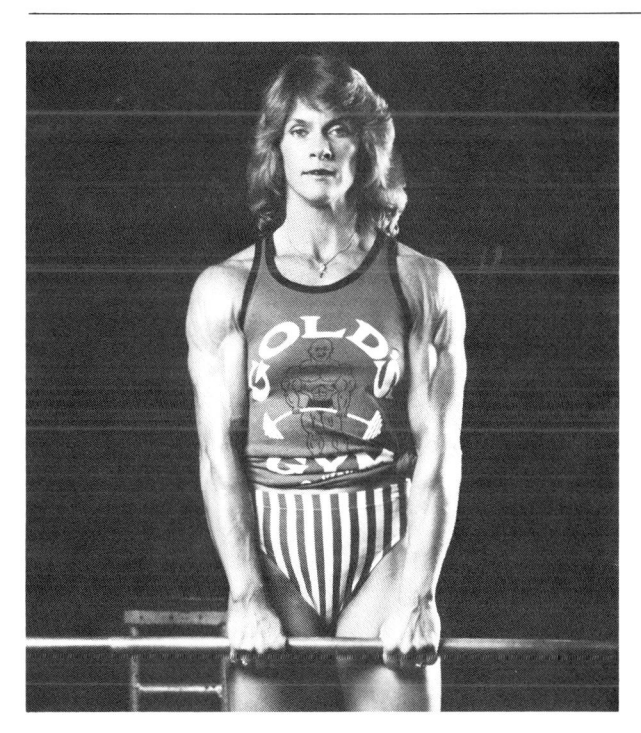

Upright Rowing—This is both a deltoid and trapezius movement. Take an overgrip in the middle of a barbell with your index fingers 4–6 inches apart. At the start of the movement you should be standing erect with your arms hanging straight down at your sides and the barbell resting across your upper thighs.

From this position, pull the barbell directly upward along the front of your body, keeping the weight 2–3 inches away from your torso. As you are pulling, your elbows should always be above your hands and wrists. Pull the bar upward until your hands contact the underside of your chin.

At this top position, your shoulders should be rotated backward as far as possible and your shoulder blades should be pressed together. Hold this top position for 2–3 seconds and then lower the weight slowly back to the starting position. Repeat the movement for the required number of repetitions.

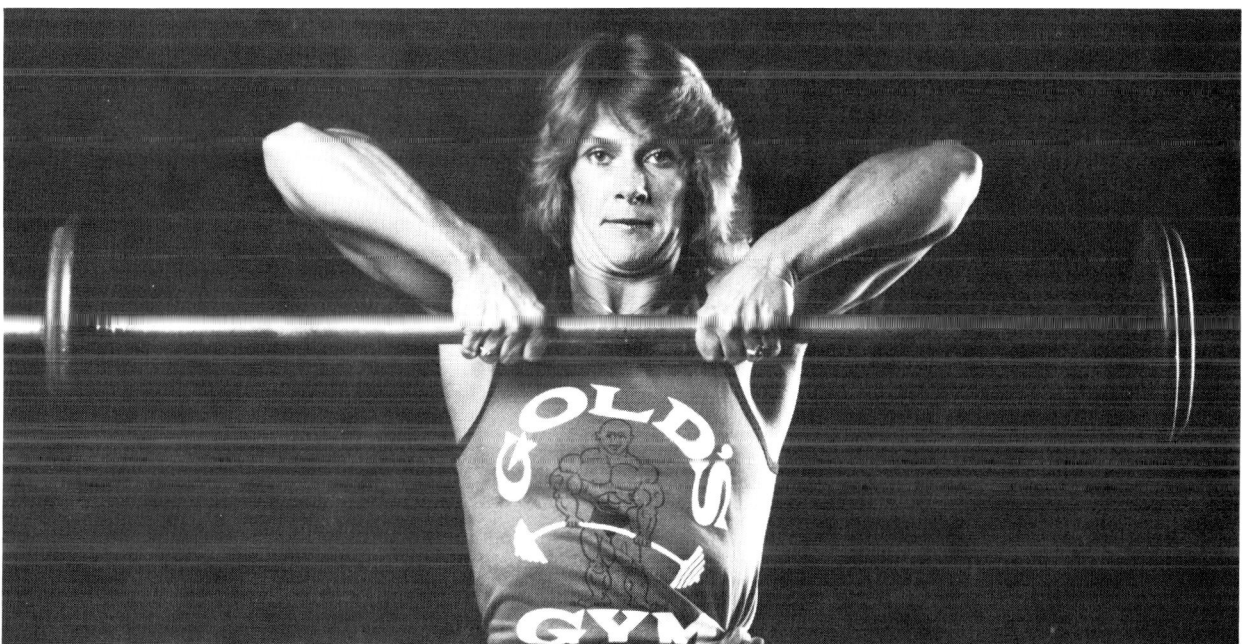

56 BODYBUILDING AND CONDITIONING FOR WOMEN

Lat Pulldowns—Similar to chinning, but less severe, in this exercise you pull the bar down to your body rather than pulling your body up to the bar. You can either sit or kneel under the lat pulley (many big gyms have a special bench with a horizontal bar; you can wedge your thighs under this bar when you do Pulldowns with a very heavy weight). You can use the same grip and hand spacing variations for Pulldowns as for Chins, and the movement is done in exactly the same manner. My personal preference for Lat Pulldowns is to do them with a narrow and reversed grip.

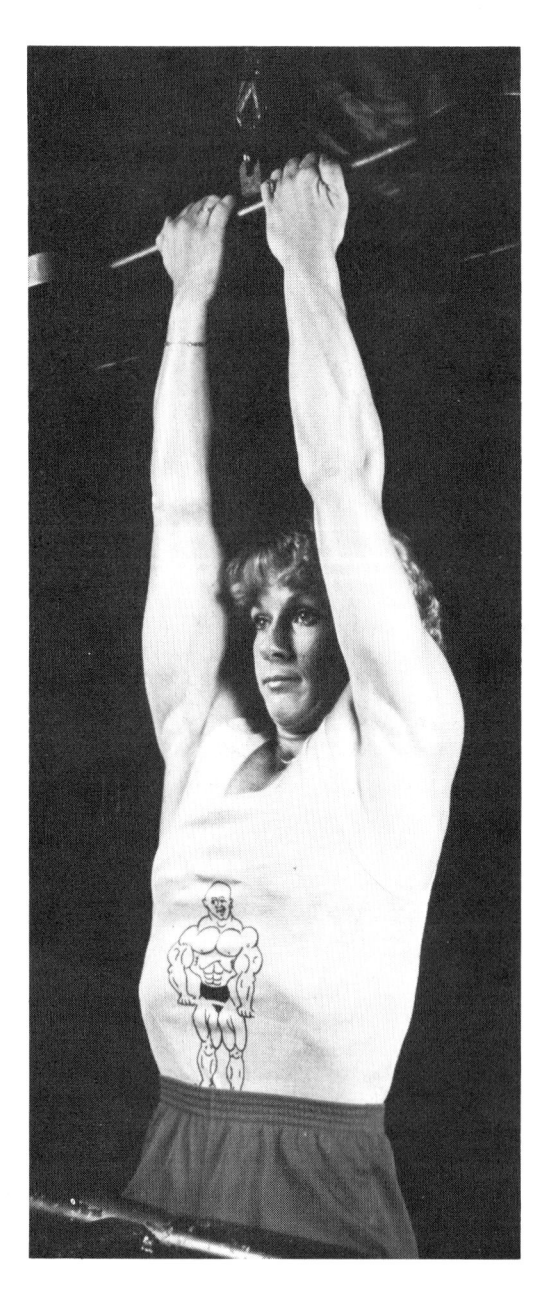

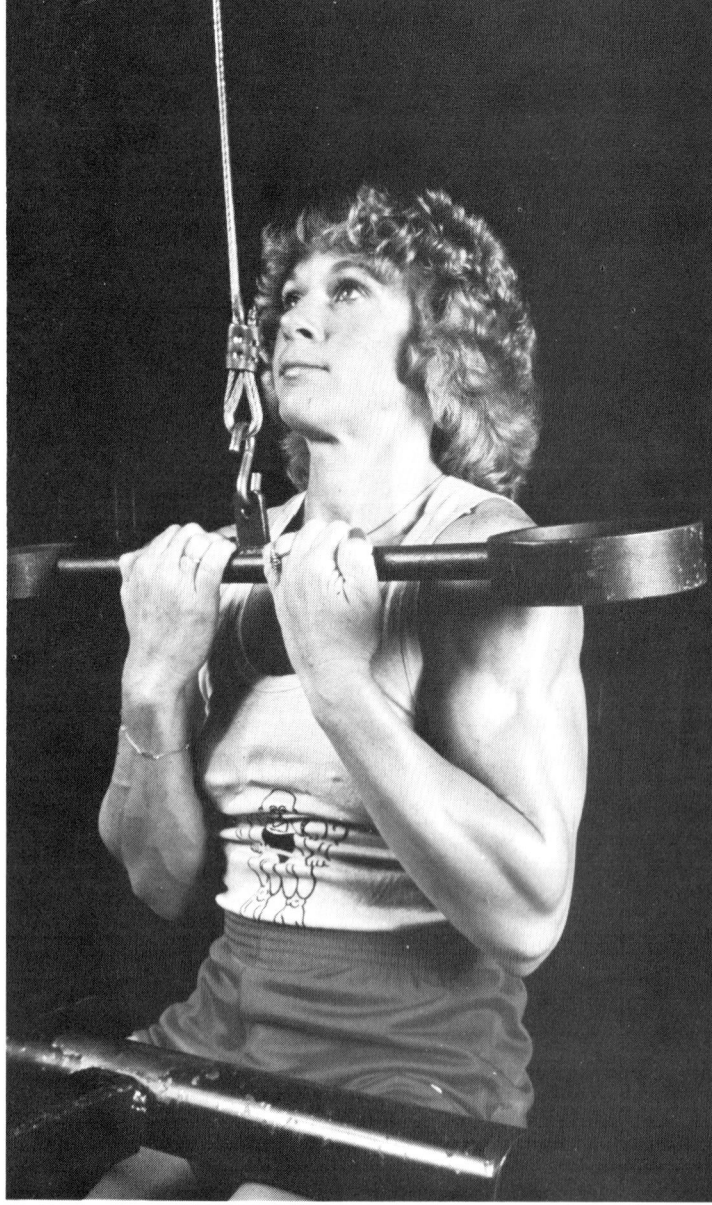

A STRONG, SENSUOUS BACK 57

Seated Pulley Rows—This variation of Bent Rowing is done with a floor pulley. While Pulley Rowing primarily stimulates the latissimus dorsi, it also strongly stresses the traps and erectors. This makes it one of the best all-round back exercises.

Sit down and brace your feet on the foot bar. Be sure your legs are kept slightly bent throughout the movement to relieve lower back strain.

Grasp the handle of the pulley, which can be either a straight bar handle or one that allows a parallel grip. I prefer the parallel-grip handle.

Begin the movement by leaning forward with your arms straight, which will fully stretch your lats. Then lean back until your torso is upright and simultaneously bend your arms until your hands touch the lower edge of your ribcage. Return to the starting point and repeat.

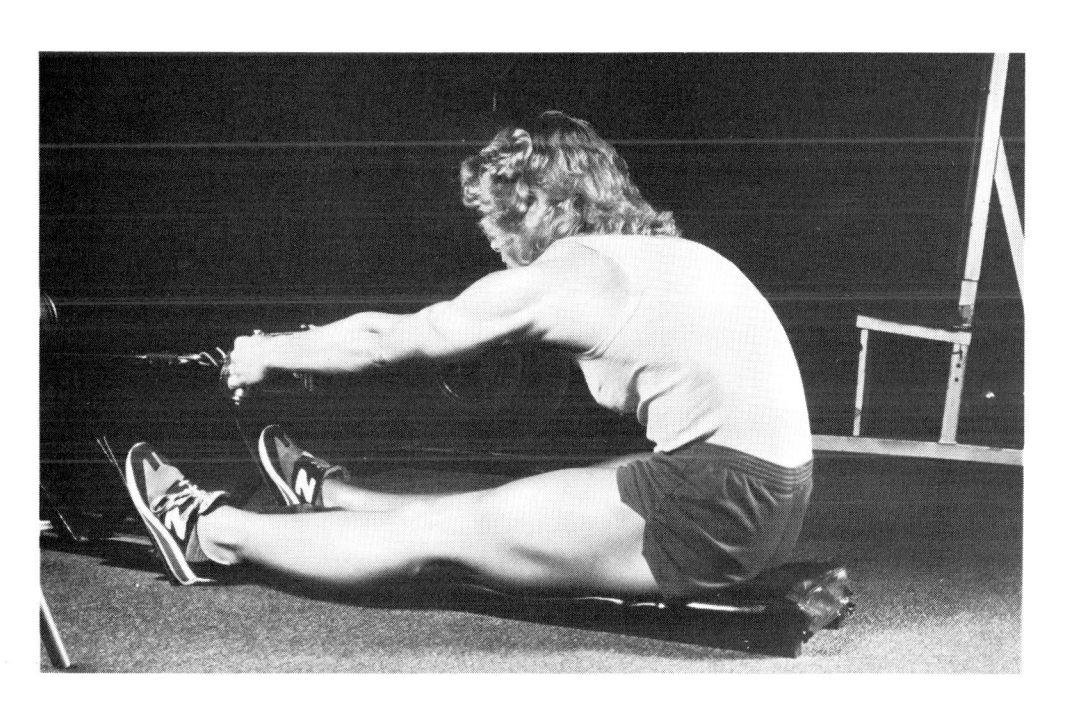

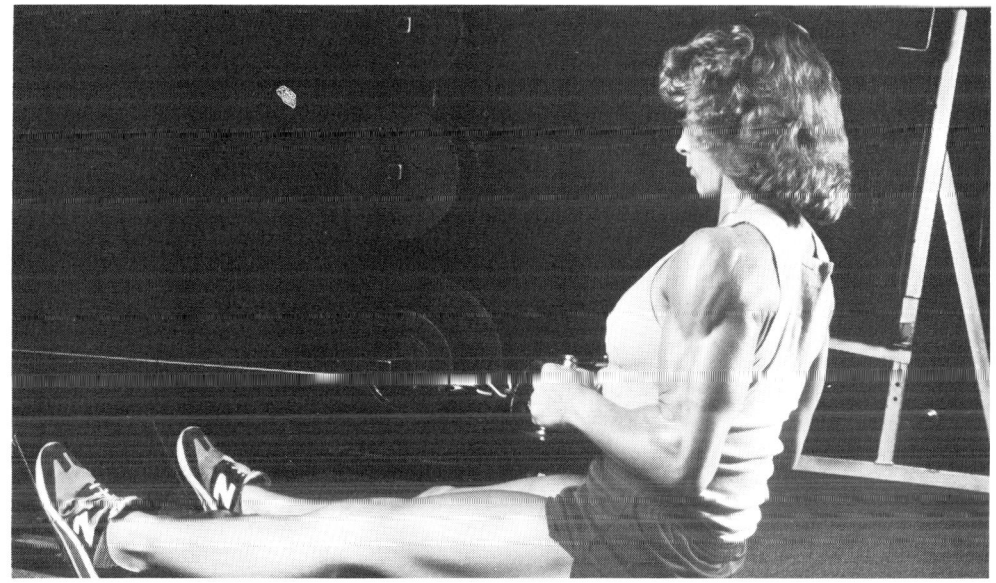

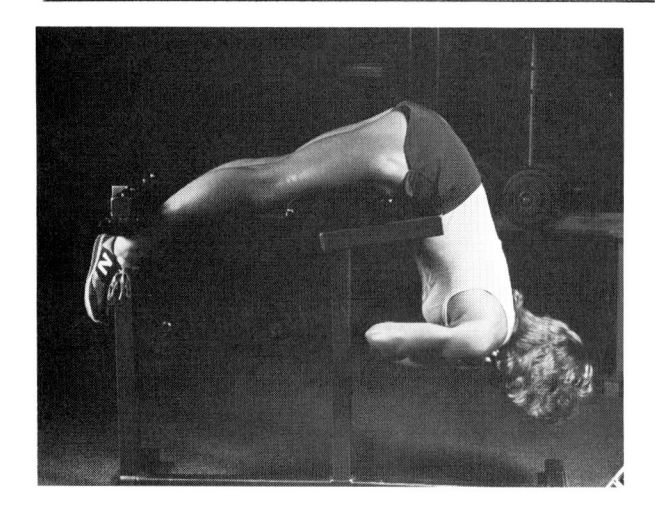

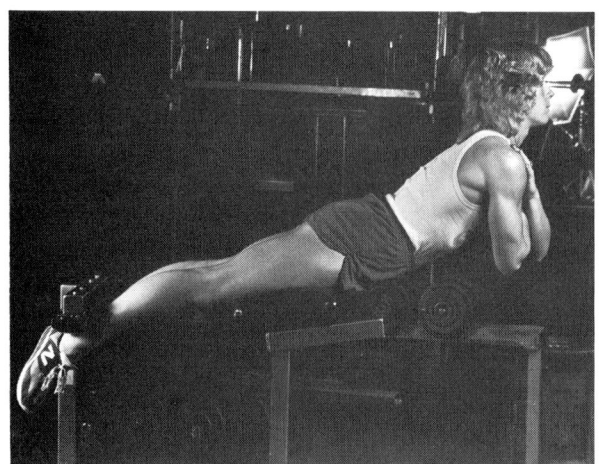

Hyperextensions—As I mentioned earlier, this is my favorite lower back exercise. It can be done either in a gym on a special Hyperextension bench or at home lying on a high table with someone holding your legs down. In either case, you should slide forward until your torso is entirely off the bench or table. When you are in the correct position, the top edge of your pelvis should be at the front edge of the table or bench pad.

Start by hanging your torso directly downward. Clasp your hands behind your neck throughout the movement. From this basic starting position, do a "Reverse Sit-Up" by arching your back and pulling your torso upward until it is slightly above an imaginary line drawn parallel to the floor. Do not arch up farther because that compresses the spinal vertebrae. Return to the starting position and repeat for the required number of repetitions.

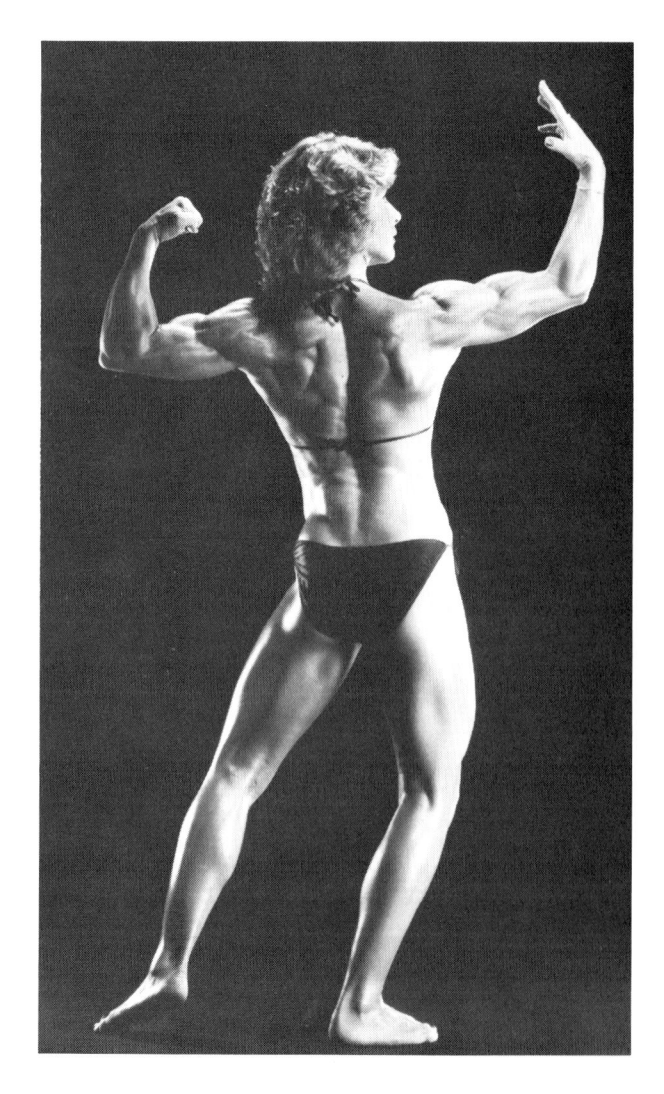

Conkwright on Posing

by Betty Weider

Lynn Conkwright is probably the best poser in women's bodybuilding. Her flawless presentation at the 1981 World Championships in Atlantic City was a major factor in her victory. And the routine she and partner Chris Dickerson put together to win the 1980 World Couples Championship was so imaginatively constructed and perfectly executed that it has set a new standard for couples posing.

"For me, putting together a good posing routine is the most enjoyable part of competitive bodybuilding," Lynn says. "What I try to do is make my routine seem almost effortless, so it just flows. But, believe me, developing a good posing routine and practicing it until you can do it perfectly is anything but easy and effortless. It requires a tremendous amount of planning and hard work."

Due to her enormous success in bodybuilding competition, Lynn is constantly being asked by beginning women bodybuilders how to go about learning to pose. Her advice is simply to begin at the beginning.

"A posing routine is made up of individual poses, so the first thing you need to know is how to do these poses. What I did was to learn each of the standard men's poses and try to modify them until I felt they were suitable for a woman. In practicing each one in front of the mirror, I would, for example, open my hand instead of making a fist, twist my body slightly to change the line, cock my hip a little—that's how I developed my favorite front double biceps pose.

"My very first posing routine didn't show much of my muscular development. I was more concerned with the movement and the flow of the posing. But in the second routine I created, I concentrated on taking a compulsory pose and putting it to music in an aesthetic way. And I made sure that I displayed all of the muscle groups to the judges, as if I were saying, 'This is how I am going to get you to look at my deltoids in a different way.' When you're posing for qualified judges, showing them your physique from a variety of angles helps them to appreciate the quality of your development."

Of course, learning each of the compulsories and the other standard poses has to be the first step. These poses are the building blocks of any routine. But they are static, and a good posing routine is anything but static. It is, Lynn believes, almost a form of dance. And for dance you need music.

"Picking the right kind of music is vital to creating a good posing routine," Lynn says. "You have to pick something that excites you, that motivates you, something you enjoy. You can't just pick any kind of music. I find that if I can feel the music, posing comes easy. Posing is like telling a story through the movement of your body, and you should be able to visualize the story that the music is telling you."

A bodybuilding routine should be good theater, Lynn believes, with dramatic tension, fast and slow parts, good dynamics and an exciting finish. Therefore, the music you choose has to have all of these things. "If your music is monotonous, your routine will be, too," she says.

"Once I have my music," explains Lynn, "I begin to construct my routine like a drama . . . with an introduction, (story) development and then a conclusion. I want a sense of completeness and wholeness in my routine, a feeling that nothing is missing. I make sure I include all of the muscular poses so that the judges will be able to see every bodypart in a flexed position. As much as a posing routine may be like dance or a gymnastics floor exercise, the sport is bodybuilding, and the judges ultimately will be looking for quality of muscle development. So you have to show them your musculature."

Lynn writes down each of the poses she has learned and practiced, then puts them in the order she wants them to go in the routine. "For example, I picked the pose I thought was my strongest and decided to begin with that. And my 'needle' pose, in which I bend all the way forward and point one leg straight up overhead, is very dramatic, so I put that right at the end. It's really a gymnastics move rather than a bodybuilding pose, but I want to show the judges that, even though I have very strong and muscular legs, I am still very flexible. Even women bodybuilders sometimes get accused of being muscle-bound."

When Lynn is certain she has all her poses in order, and has a story with a beginning, middle and end, she begins to establish transitional moves and connecting poses.

"Rhythm is very important to a bodybuilding routine. You don't want the judges to feel that the music is going on while you're just standing still. I don't consider the connecting poses true bodybuilding poses; they're smooth, fluid movements that let me flow from one bodybuilding pose to another. This is very much like a gymnastics floor exercise where you do many graceful movements between the compulsory tumbling movements."

Lynn feels that her gymnastics background has been a tremendous help to her in bodybuilding. For one thing, the strenuous training she subjected herself to for so many years is the basis of the championship physique she has today. And the grace, balance and performing experience she acquired from years of competition have contributed immensely to that sense of perfection and polish she exhibits onstage.

"Women's gymnastics is really four sports, since there are four different events, and I used to train one to two hours a day for each one. Even when I went to college, school was secondary to training. But all that training taught me about hard work and discipline, and I have applied myself to bodybuilding with the same dedication."

Lynn Conkwright begins planning and practicing her posing routine months before a contest, going over the movements again and again, changing and improving the routine wherever necessary, until she can perform each movement with absolute precision. However, as far as she is concerned, a routine is never finished, never perfect. There is always room for improvement and she works at making her routine better every single day.

"A routine should be balanced," she says, "in some poses you should face one way, in others you should face another. There should be front, side and back poses, graceful poses and muscular ones. The judges have already seen the compulsory poses, seen your body in a static mode, so the purpose of the routine is to show them your body in a fluid way, to demonstrate how the muscles function and interact with one another, to demonstrate the true beauty of muscles in motion.

"For example, I don't do a standard lat spread in my routine, but I have three different poses that show my lats from various angles. Twisting, from the side, and so on. Or I try to show off my calves different ways . . . in a standing pose and a kneeling one. And I'm always looking for new poses. I study photos of other women bodybuilders and say, 'Ah, that looks nice,' and then I try to understand how she got that effect. I learn a lot from magazines like *Muscle & Fitness*, studying the photos and figuring out what each pose shows and why it works for certain bodybuilders."

But Lynn doesn't just learn from other bodybuilders. She also studies dancers, gymnasts and others who can show her a new way of demonstrating the dynamics of the body or inspire her to add a new movement to her routine. "I never wait until I am ready to enter a contest before working on my posing," she says.

CONKWRIGHT ON POSING 61

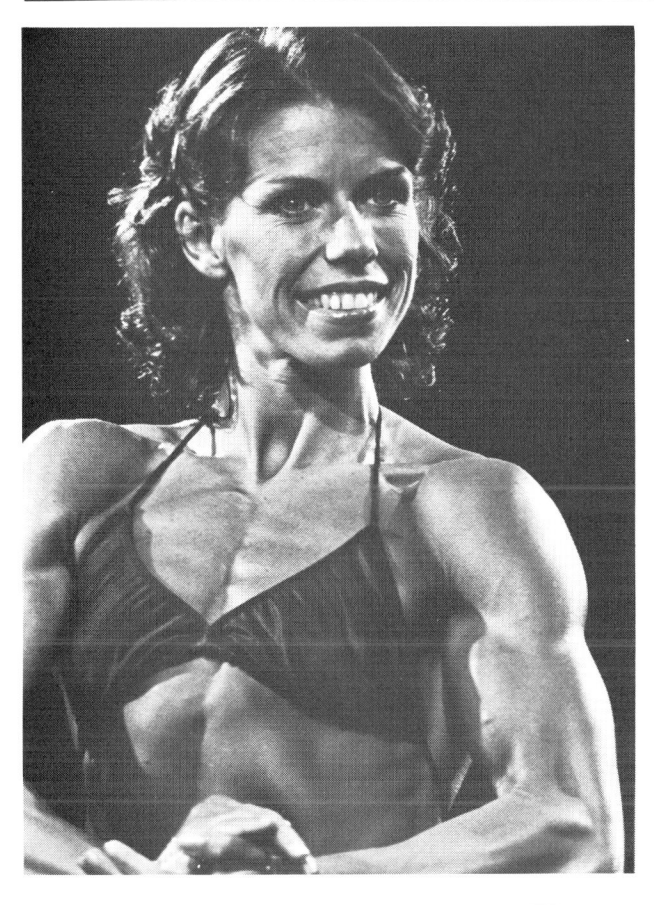

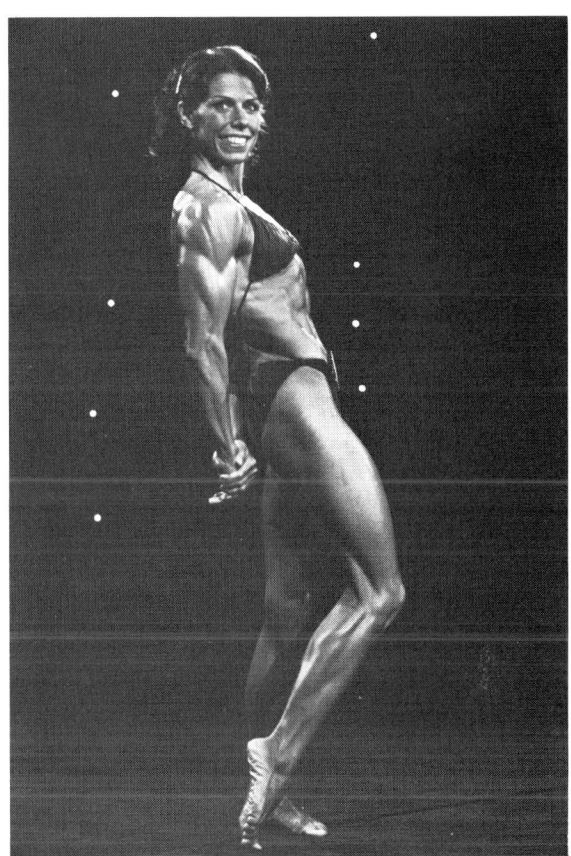

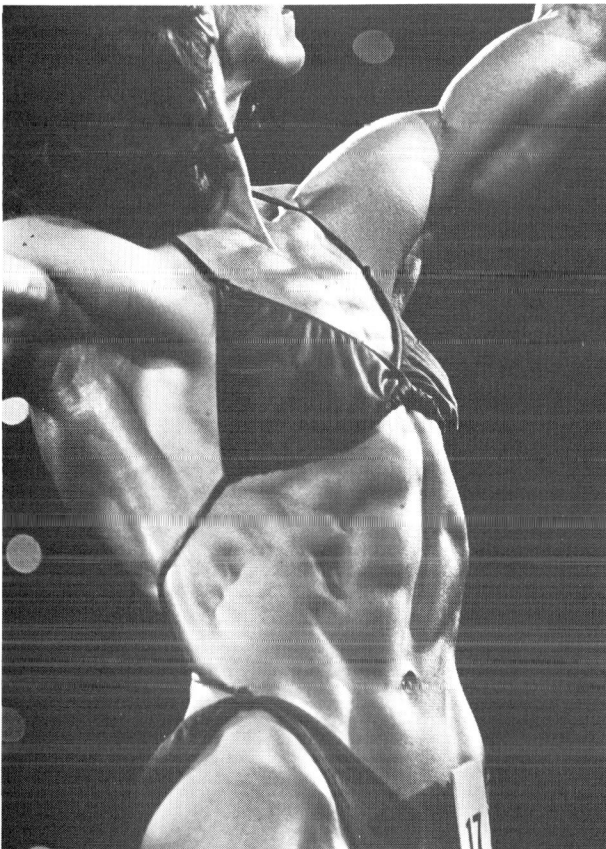

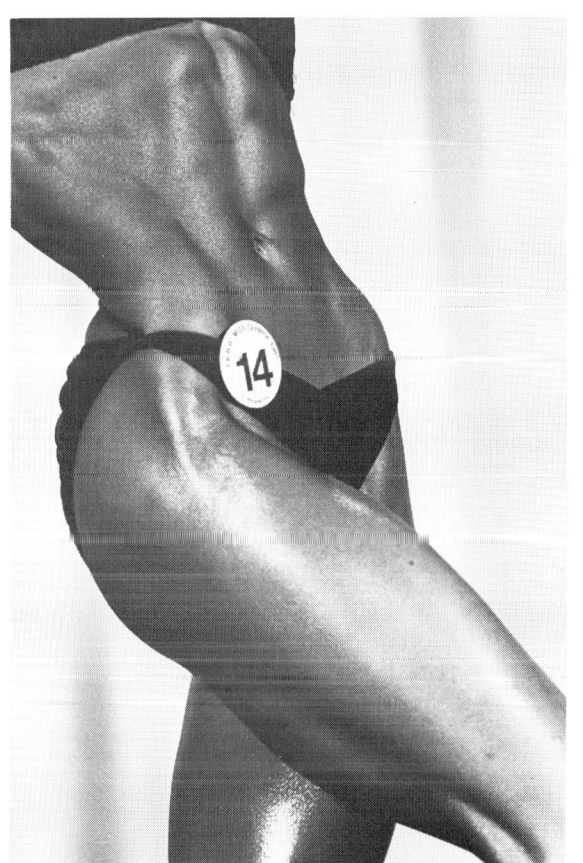

"I am constantly thinking about it, working on it, analyzing it and rehearsing."

Lynn believes that the quality of her posing routine comes about mainly due to two factors: 1. She plans and composes her routine very carefully, spending weeks and months putting it together just the way she wants; and 2. She spends months and months in long hours of practice and rehearsal to make her execution absolutely flawless.

"After each contest, I work on my routine and try to improve it. Actually, I have four different pieces of music I can use, depending on the effect I want to create. The aim of a good posing routine is to create an emotional response in the judges—they have already looked at your physique from a technical point of view—and the music you use, plus the way you match your poses to the music, are what you use to make them respond the way you want."

One of Lynn's greatest fans—understandably—is her posing partner Chris Dickerson, who's considered a master poser in his own right. When he was looking for a new posing partner last year, he considered all the top women bodybuilders. He chose Lynn for one reason: he thought she was the best.

"Lynn is diligent and hard working in practice, every bit as much a perfectionist as I am, and she's the perfect partner onstage. We both approach posing from the same point of view—a routine should have a story, a theme. The routine we put together for Atlantic City was a blend of my talents and hers, with both of us contributing ideas. And I feel it was highly successful. If you want to see women's posing at its best, you don't have to look any further than Lynn. She's tremendous!"

Rachel McLish: "Variety Is My Spice of Life"

by Bill Reynolds

"Variety is the mother of enjoyment."
—Benjamin Disraeli

"There's nothing new about the idea of injecting maximum variety into bodybuilding workouts," Rachel McLish told me with a smile that would melt the heart of the most jaded journalist.

"The human body adapts very quickly to any external stimulus—high reps, low reps, heavy weights, light weights, high-fat foods, low-fat foods, varying sleep patterns, different types of aerobic workouts. It even adapts to certain kinds of makeup, shampoos and hair conditioners.

"Muscles grow larger and stronger when they are stressed with a heavier weight than they are accustomed to handling, but they very quickly adapt to this new weight. They also adapt to a particular workout. By constantly changing my workouts, however, I am able to keep my muscles off-balance. I shock them so they can't adapt to a consistent stress and they're forced to grow larger and stronger. I *never* allow my muscles to adapt to a set type of workload. Essentially, I follow a sort of 'nonroutine routine,' and it works!"

Like most bodybuilders, Rachel has a set off-season goal—to improve her overall proportion, symmetry and muscle mass. "Then during my precontest cycle," she says, "I put the finishing touches on my physique, sharpening and polishing all the new muscular development I've acquired during my off-season training. I'm talking about the finest and most minute details of muscular definition that I can't pay attention to in the off-season."

OFF-SEASON vs PRECONTEST VARIANTS

"Prior to competition I'll train six days per week, but in the off-season I'll work out only four days a week, and I'll postpone a scheduled training session for a day when I find that I can't give a workout 100% of my energy and concentration. Off-season I'll train each muscle group—even calves and abdominals—twice per week, because I can recuperate best on such a four-day split routine. Without full recuperation, it's difficult to add muscle mass to your physique.

"In my precontest phase I still work most of my muscle groups twice per week. The exception is abdominals, which I train up to six days each week. I rest a little less between sets prior to a competition, but I don't really monitor my rest intervals that closely. Speed isn't an intensity factor in my workouts, because I prefer to obtain my exercise intensity from using heavy weights with strong mental concentration during each set.

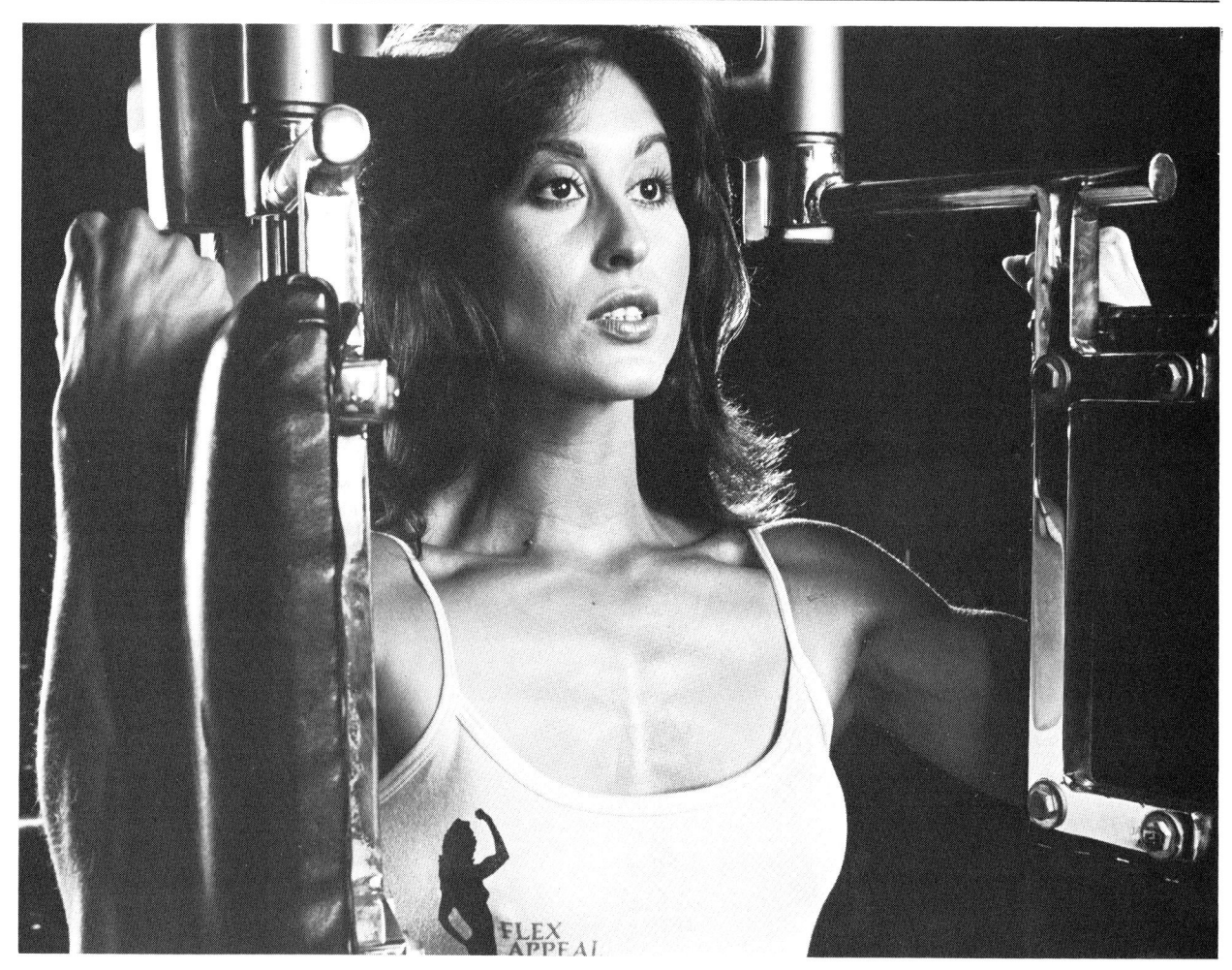

"On days when I have things to do or am feeling especially energetic I'll zip through a workout. At other times, however, I prefer a more moderate pace that allows me to get optimally psyched up for each set. Then my workouts take a bit longer."

Rachel's training methods and workouts are fairly similar during both cycles, but she feels markedly stronger in the off-season, due to these three factors:

1. Her diet is more relaxed, so she has more energy than when following a precontest diet.

2. She isn't doing as much aerobic training, which also improves the amount of energy she has available for each workout.

3. She is not as concerned with injuring herself, so she's able to go all-out with heavy poundages virtually every workout.

"Prior to a competition, I tend to hold back in my training," Rachel revealed. "I don't need a joint or muscle injury when a contest is coming up, and I feel that this is when I'm most prone to injury. Most bodybuilders with whom I've talked also feel that they're most susceptible to injury when their energy reserves are low close to a show."

SETS, REPS PER BODYPART

I asked Miss Olympia about the total number of sets she does for each bodypart. She answered, "Except for my abdominals, I do basically the same number of sets for each muscle group prior to a competition as I do in the off-season. For large muscle groups (back, chest and thighs) I'll do twelve sets, for triceps nine, and for biceps and calves six. I hit abs with ten-twelve sets each workout in the off-season and twelve-fifteen prior to a contest.

"Generally speaking, I do less total sets for a bodypart than most serious women bodybuilders, but I am sure that my intensity within each set is higher than average. I always try to make every set count.

"My thighs and calves come up very easily, but I still do plenty of high-intensity sets for them to achieve hardness and detail. Many women with naturally big thighs mistakenly stop exercising them. They'd be better off training them hard, because you *must* keep overloading them to give the thighs shape and quality. I just work my legs with higher-than-normal reps—12–15 in the off-season and 15–20 prior to a contest—to keep them from becoming too massive.

"My forearms also respond quickly, particularly because I play a lot of racquetball. Rather than increasing the reps on my forearm exercises, however, I do fewer total sets, normally no more than three or four each workout. So, you can see that you have alternative ways to treat strong muscle groups—perform higher reps, or do less total sets."

Rachel normally keeps her reps—except for thighs and abdominals—in the 6–8 range in the off-season and up to 10–12 prior to competing. And, during the workouts we've taken together, I've observed that virtually every repetition is of very high quality. At times she'll do forced reps, while at others she does a lot of burns to push her muscles past the point of failure. These burns are partial reps with a range of motion only six to eight inches, usually in peak contraction.

"Peak contraction reps and burns are particularly effective for building muscle mass and quality," the current World Professional Champion added. "But in harmony with my philosophy of injecting a maximum degree of variety into my training, this also changes from workout to workout. Going past the point of normal muscular failure with forced reps or burns is fine, but I certainly don't push all my sets that far. Remember, keep your muscles off-balance, and they'll keep growing.

"I also like to do supersets, especially when there is a time factor and I have to get a workout over as quickly as I can without sacrificing intensity. I particularly like to perform pre-exhaustion supersets. Typical pre-exhaustion exercise groupings include Side Laterals with Overhead Presses, Cable Crossovers with Decline Presses and Leg Extensions with Squats or Leg Presses."

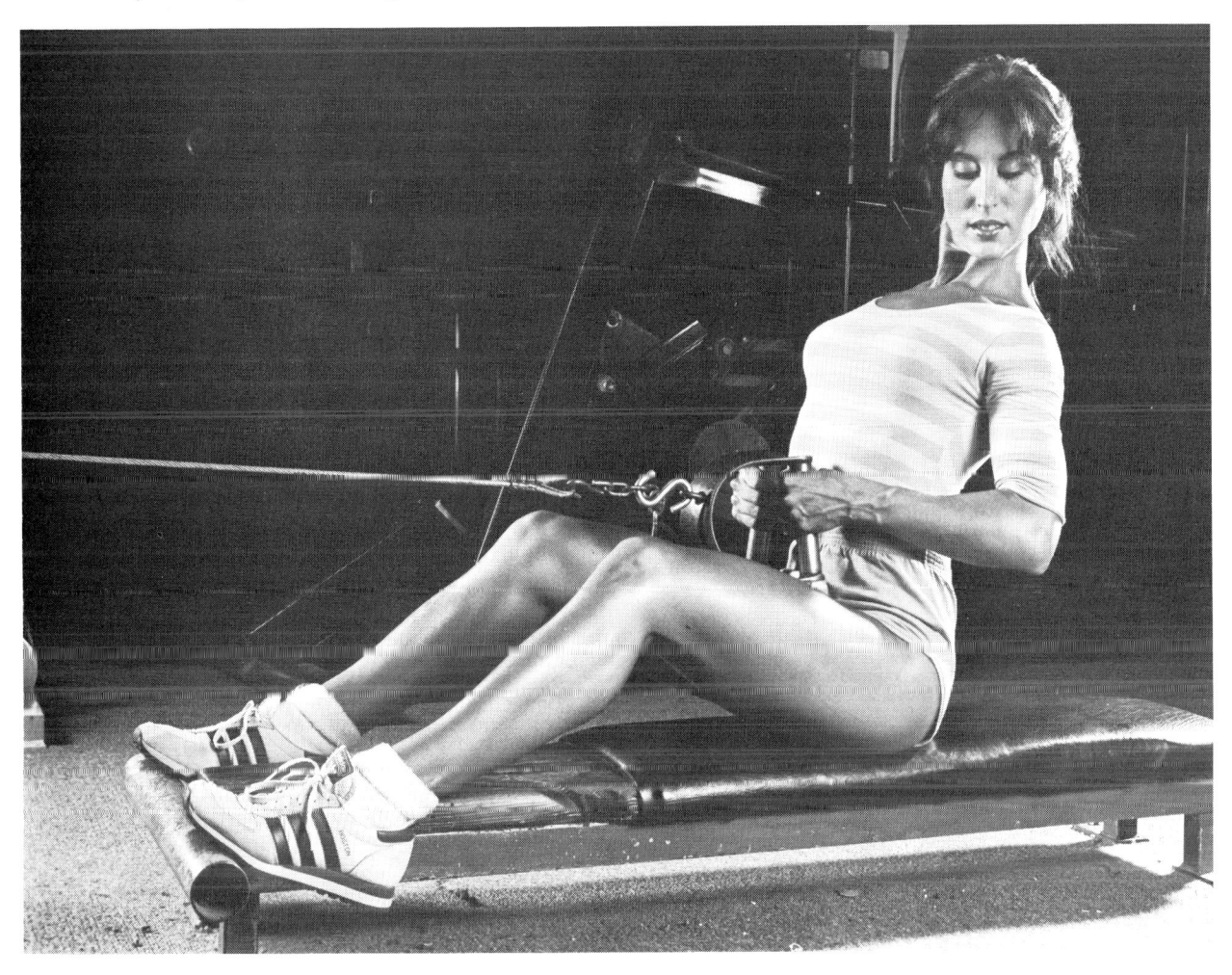

THE MOST FROM TECHNIQUE

I've noticed that Rachel injects variety into her workouts not only through choice of exercises, but also through uniquely different methods of doing each exercise. When I asked her to explain why she performed each exercise differently, her answer was typically insightful and clear.

"The reason can be boiled down to three words—*muscle contraction specificity*. You must do a movement a particular way if you want to achieve a predetermined appearance of the muscle it affects.

"If you place your feet wide apart as you do Squats, for example, it stresses the inner thigh muscles, particularly higher up, while a narrow stance hits the central section and outer sweep of the quads. Doing Squats with your toes angled outward places stronger stress on the *vastus medialis* muscle on the inside of your thigh just above the knees. Done with your toes pointed slightly inward, Squats stress the lower and outer sections of your thighs.

"Such performance variations exist for virtually every exercise, and I do every possible variation in my workouts, particularly prior to a competition. Then, I want to hit a muscle group from every possible angle to promote complete development. At other times, I proceed in accordance with my muscle contraction specificity principle—I most frequently use the performance variation of an exercise that stresses the part of a muscle that most needs additional development."

I asked Rachel how she learned all these exercise performance variations.

"I've learned over more than six years of steady training and experimentation exactly which method hits every part of my physique, just as every aspiring woman bodybuilder must. I used to spend up to 15 hours a day working in the Sport Palace of Harlingen, Texas, and I didn't want to become bored. So I filled my unoccupied time by experimenting with every possible exercise on each available piece of equipment.

"Very few women realize that I have so many years of training and *learning* behind me. All the years you put into your training can yield so much more when you consciously use your brain to get the most out of each exercise. Think about how you can do a movement differently to achieve a different muscle contraction specificity in the area it works, and in the long run you'll be light years ahead of the bodybuilders who don't."

I asked Rachel if she practiced ISO-Tension contraction during her precontest preparation phase.

"Yes, and it's resulted in a marked improvement in my muscle quality," she answered. "I do a high number of hard repetition muscle flexes each day, both between sets in a workout and at odd times of the day—driving my car, grocery shopping, at dinner and

---

TRAINING TIPS FROM MISS OLYMPIA

- If you feel like missing a workout, you should at least get in your car and drive to the gym. Do five light sets and walk out; you'll be farther ahead than if you had remained at home. Do high reps, and play on new machines as if they were toys. Sometimes this results in a great workout. If it doesn't, go home, relax, drink a glass of wine and take up the next day where you left off.
- Be observant and open to new knowledge. I personally gain something from everyone I meet. Even if a person is a bum, he can teach me something.
- Keep a detailed training and nutrition diary. It's the best way of making sense of the confusing array of information and techniques that confront any bodybuilder. I write down everything—every set I do, every morsel I consume, how I look to myself, how I feel, and every other bit of info I feel might have an effect on my bodybuilding.
- I could care less what I weigh. What counts is the *quality* of muscular development. I've weighed 118 and looked fat, and I've weighed 123 and been in great shape. The judges don't weigh you, so your weight is irrelevant. To be a winner you have to keep the muscle mass up and the fat down.
- Don't be afraid to sweat. I like the feeling of sweating during an all-out workout. Sweating is very good for you—it cleanses your body of toxins from the inside out. There's nothing unfeminine about sweat during a bodybuilding workout.

—Rachel McLish

whenever else I think of it. I believe that any woman can harden up and gain better control of her muscles if she uses ISO-Tension consistently when peaking for a competition."

AEROBICS IN TRAINING

My last question on training was how much aerobic exercise Rachel included in her daily training schedule. She answered, "Aerobic workouts are an essential facet of my training philosophy, although it took me a while to realize their importance. Prior to my first competition, I had been teaching aerobic dance classes, and I was very tight-looking as a result. After I really got into bodybuilding, however, I did less and less aerobic training.

"When I began meeting all the champs I'd read so much about in *Muscle & Fitness*, I learned many new training techniques from them. This led to a series of experiments, during which I neglected my aerobics, which in turn made it more difficult to get cut up for a competition. This past year, however, I've gone back to doing more aerobic classes.

"During a defining phase, I increase my aerobic activity, doing at least a solid two hours of aerobics, and often up to three hours. I tend to stick to playing racquetball, taking aerobic classes, cycling and running, and of course I rotate these aerobic activities from day to day. For best results I also need variety in my aerobic sessions."

The closer a competition, the more crucial diet becomes, but Rachel is no fanatic: "I do enough aerobic training that I never need to go under 1500 calories per day, even prior to competing. It took me a long time to understand that I have to *eat* to have both mass and quality onstage. And this realization has been a key factor in my improvement recently."

PEAKING THROUGH SACRIFICE

"Last year I fasted a lot when preparing for competition. I lost all my bodyfat this way, but I also had to sacrifice a great deal of lean body mass because I wasn't eating enough to support a proper degree of muscle mass. I got ripped up through fasting, but I didn't have the fullness and shapeliness of muscle mass that I need to appear at my best."

Rachel even drinks wine during a contest preparation phase: "It's good for relaxation, and I really enjoy quality white wines and champagne. You really don't have to sacrifice that much in getting ready for a contest *if* you go about it intelligently.

"A number of bodybuilders monitor their water balances, but I like to play with mine in the days leading up to a competition. When you are on a low-salt diet all the time, your body will adapt to it and respond in an exaggerated manner by retaining a great deal of water any time you take in a little salt. Having learned this, I ate a ton of salt a week before the last Olympia. I would drink a margarita and eat potato chips and pizza, and I was bloated.

"Because I was bloated with water, no one who saw me a week before the Olympia could believe I was entering. Then for a couple of days before the show I monitored my salt intake very closely, and my body released all of the water it had been holding. By tricking my body this way, I ended up looking very tight and muscular."

Rachel is a closet chocoholic, but never abuses her body by eating junk food without a purpose. "I have occasional cravings," she confessed, "and they are usually a good indication that my body requires the nutrients I crave. Yesterday I ate three scoops of chocolate ice cream, and when I reviewed my diary notes, I saw that I consumed very little fat over the previous four days. My body was craving the fats in ice cream."

In answer to my question about supplement usage, Rachel replied, "I'm a firm believer in *over*-supplementation, but only in the water-soluble vitamins and minerals. I don't supplement my diet with extra A, D, E, or K, the oil-soluble vitamins, but I take in plenty of B vitamins, C and chelated minerals."

MENTAL INTENSITY

Turning to the mental aspect of bodybuilding, Rachel told me that she has a very clear vision of how she wants her physique to ultimately appear: "Because I can visualize a part of my physique much more easily than the whole, I like to think of only one or two bodyparts. Usually, I visualize primarily those muscle groups that I feel are weak in the manner I'd like them to soon appear. When I spot a lagging bodypart, I become almost obsessed with bringing it up.

"Or I occasionally pick on something that isn't up to par—such as my posing now—and I give it intense attention. It's only prior to a competition that I can maintain everything at a high pitch, but even then I can go at this accelerated pace only for a few weeks before faltering."

Rachel also has a very rational approach to goal setting: "If you think of something too mind-boggling—such as winning a major international competition—you probably won't achieve it. I've found it best to break my long-term goals into smaller, short-range goals.

"I used to become discouraged occasionally because I was gaining muscle mass so slowly, as is the case with most women bodybuilders. Now I prefer to train for quality development rather than pure mass because the mass will ultimately come if I follow this approach."

This concept is similar to something Frank Zane recently told me: "Regardless of how negative something like losing a competition seems at the time, you can turn it into positive energy. A loss just gives me greater incentive to keep training hard."

"I can agree with that," Rachel smiled. "Losing the '81 Olympia was one of the best things that could have happened to me because reliving the experience has given me so much drive, enthusiasm and training energy that it's pushed me to new heights of development. Also, an occasional loss keeps a bodybuilder from getting too cocky.

"Rex Dante, my memory dynamics teacher, called this process 'turning the dial.' You turn a negative experience into something positive. I'm a firm believer that everything happens to you for a purpose."

Rachel McLish's final mental technique involves psyching herself up before each workout: "On the way to the gym I think about a variety of things that give me greater drive.

"Often good rock music will do it. At other times I get psyched up by listening to classical music or my inspirational religious cassette tapes or by thinking about my competitors and how good they are. And, I sometimes think about my parents, all they've done for me over the years, and how it's now my turn to give them something back.

"All these methods work in rotation, and the variety is again important. The mind can also quickly adapt to a certain psyching stimulus and become inured to it, so you should never stick to any one psyching method."

ASSUMING A SUCCESSFUL POSE

As hinted earlier, Rachel feels that she needs much more work on her posing. "Believe me, I haven't begun to tap my potential. I used to dance in public, practicing for hours every day and loving every minute of it, and I'm sure I can do the same with my posing.

"For most of the year I ignore my entire routine, working instead on short series of poses. I get comfortable with moving from pose to pose—regardless of sequence—so I can look fluid onstage even if I deviate from my set routine. This way I can improvise a routine if something happens onstage to interrupt my normal program.

"One of the most exciting aspects of posing is that, as my body becomes more completely developed, I can do many poses that I couldn't pull off previously. For example, it's only in the past few months that I've been able to do a good three-quarters back shot.

"I'm careful to watch all the contestants at each show when I guest pose to pick up ideas. I was in Trinidad recently, and they posed spectacularly there, incorporating theatrics and facial expressions into their routines. Some of the things I learned there will be included in my future routines."

As our interview drew to a close, I noticed that Rachel had thick calluses on each hand.

"I'm proud of them," she laughed. "Many people seem to have the idea that I don't train hard. Calluses are an integral part of bodybuilding, and they verify the fact that I train extremely hard and use very heavy weights in my workouts."

With her unique combination of femininity and muscular development, Rachel McLish has shown how a woman bodybuilder should look. We couldn't have chosen a better person to bear the standard of the new women's sport.□

Energy:
Keep Yours at Muscle-Building Levels

by Raymond Schuessler

The Porsche 928 is a highly sophisticated piece of machinery. To keep it working at optimal levels, you've got to feed it high-octane fuel and then run it as its maker intended. If not, the auto becomes just another sluggish heap on the road, suffering routine breakdowns that cost a fortune to repair.

That's not unlike the human body—the most complex machine ever created. In order to keep it working at peak efficiency, it must be maintained precisely. And at the core of an effective maintenance program are proper nourishment and demanding exercise, both of which supply the body with all-important energy.

Those who succeed in any area of endeavor have an abundance of energy. Achievers are typically alert, confident and quick to take advantage of an opportunity. Success becomes their habit because of these attributes, which spring from an energetic, well-conditioned mind and body.

Look at the activities of anyone who has achieved a high level of performance in a given field; you will invariably witness extraordinary outputs of both physical and mental energy. And those who originally had the ability and talent to succeed but didn't fell by the wayside for the simple reason they tired easily. They couldn't quite make that last mile, so to speak.

Bodybuilding peak performer Tom Platz, Mr. Universe and top Mr. Olympia contender, is literally a human dynamo. Whether you walk in on one of Tom's workouts or one of his enormously popular motivational seminars, the atmosphere is crackling with electricity. And the confidence Tom exudes stems from his knowledge that if and when he needs that extra energy it is there for his summoning.

Winston Churchill's life included enough activity to make five men famous. When he was in his 70s, he swam regularly, was inordinately fond of boating and in one period of political eclipse he interspersed oil painting with the manual labor of masonry at his country place. To Churchill (as to many superior people), life was activity. He believed in the rule that you are living best and most when you are active.

Why is it peak performers are endowed with so much extra energy? Was it a lucky accident of birth that Tom Platz ended up a highly charged, motivated individual? Did Winston Churchill draw his inspiration from some divine source?

In reality there is nothing mystical about the source of that fuel which turns life into what William Blake called "a joyous dance of energy." As is the case with anything of value worth acquiring and keeping, we must choose to make the effort that leads to the acquisition of energy.

One medical doctor summed it up by saying,

"The best antidote to fatigue is to get tired more often—the more often you get physically tired, the more you build up your energy quotient. It's as simple as that."

It is an axiom that muscles which are not used will waste away. And once your body starts wasting away so will your energy, your sex drive, your business and social success—your life.

The overwhelming weight of medical evidence points to the fact that all of the body's systems, including our minds, require regular, vigorous exercise. Countless experiments have proved that exercise will increase strength, stamina and flexibility. It will make you look, feel and work better and serve to enhance the quality of your life.

All physicians agree that positive health benefits, both physical and mental, result from regular exercise. We are really what our muscles make us—weak or strong, vigorous or lethargic. And, in turn, we either advance in our work or apathetically remain where we are.

Before embarking on any physical training program, we at the Weider Research Clinic recommend you visit a doctor for a complete physical checkup. There are possible medical reasons for fatigue which should be dispelled before you take up training of any kind. A heart defect, for instance, can slow circulation. An underactive thyroid gland can cause sluggishness. Creeping diabetes can disturb metabolism and result in fatigue. Most likely no medical problem will be found, but it is best to be sure.

Research from the Washington University School of Medicine shows that lack of exercise is one of the factors responsible for a person's being too tired to exercise in the first place. Dr. John C. Hollozy explains that exercise increases the efficiency of the heart system and the muscles in using oxygen.

By the way, if you think that 5–10 minutes of light calisthenics a day is sufficient exercise, forget it. Vigorous exercise must be performed continuously for 30 minutes or more to be of any benefit. You must huff and puff a bit, and work up a sweat.

Why is exercise so effective in upping our energy quotient? A quick look at some simple exercise physiology will provide the answer. Every one of our voluntary muscles is surrounded by a network of capillaries to supply its fuel needs during work. Exercise not only draws more blood to the muscle, it also aids in the movement of blood. As a muscle functions

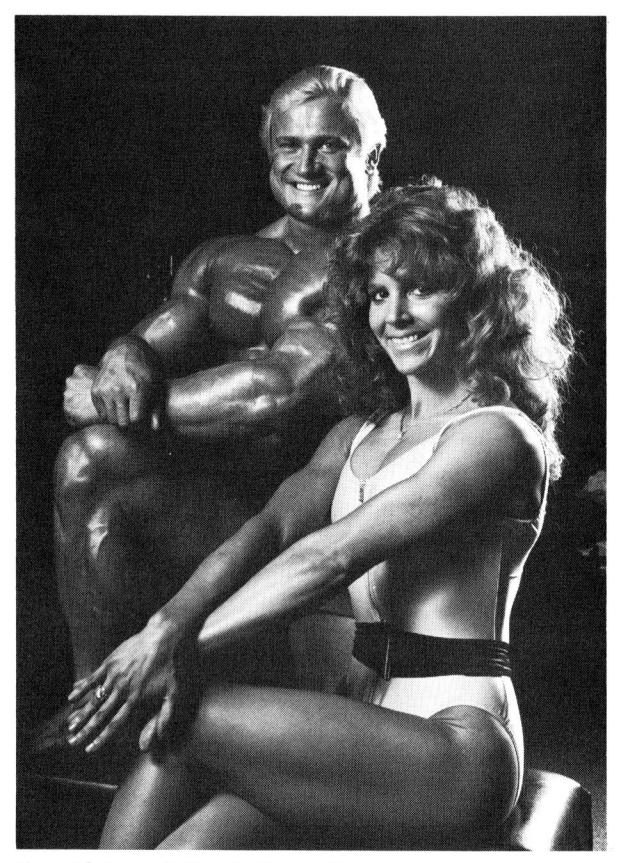

Tom Platz and Candy Csencsits.

by contracting (or reducing its length), it literally squeezes the blood out of the capillaries into the larger veins, thus making more room for the influx of oxygen-laden blood from the arteries.

When you don't exercise, the tiny, web-like capillaries which feed the muscles don't get enough blood, causing the muscles and other tissues to weaken. It's important to understand that the bloodstream carries food and oxygen to every cell of the body and, in turn, takes away waste material. When this system functions optimally, we live more vigorously, contract fewer illnesses and are more resistant to the wear and tear of stress.

When formulating an exercise program it is essential that you provide direct stimulation to the six major muscle masses of the body. Only weight resistance exercise can accomplish this effectively. Those six major areas are the thighs, back, chest, shoulders, arms and abdomen. Stimulating these muscle masses with weight resistance exercise every other day will aid significantly in maintaining superb health and vigor later in life.

There are many exercises that work two or more muscles simultaneously, and thus help in economizing your time. Chins, for instance, work the latissimus of the back along with the biceps on the front of the upper arm. Push-Ups work the pecs (or chest muscles) and the triceps on the back of the upper arm. The exercises should be arranged in order of the size of the muscle they activate, starting with the largest muscles first, working down to the smallest. Starting with the largest muscles, the thighs, we would then proceed to work the back, the chest, the shoulders, arms and then waist. Before getting into the vigorous portion of the workout, it's essential to warm up the body as a whole to cut down on the likelihood of injury. The routine below begins with two warm-up exercises, and then follows with exercises for the major masses (in descending order of muscle size). Do only one set of each exercise.

1. Jumping Jacks—15 reps.
2. Dumbbell Swings—15 reps.
3. Squats—12 reps.
4. Lunges—12 reps.
5. Barbell Cleans—12 reps.
6. Push-Ups—12 reps.
7. Bench Press—12 reps.
8. Barbell Press—12 reps.
9. Dumbbell Curls—12 reps.
10. Leg Raises on Chinning Bar—12 reps.

Those just getting started in weight training should not exceed the suggested number of sets and reps for at least a month. It is important to develop a baseline capacity before attempting anything more demanding. Choose a weight for the two warm-up exercises that allow 15 easy repetitions. For the remaining eight exercises, choose a weight that allows you to perform the suggested 12 repetitions, with the last rep being mildly difficult. After a month or so on this program, you can add a second set to each exercise, including the warm-up exercises. Again, perform the first set with a weight that allows you to finish the 12th rep with a little difficulty—the 12th rep should not require an all-out effort! Keep the weight the same for the second set, but this time, rather than stopping at any prescribed number of reps, continue the set until you can't perform one more rep no matter how hard you try! Rest no more than two minutes between sets unless you're feeling light-headed or nauseous. Over a period of time, however, make a consistent effort to cut the rest time between sets. This will help develop your cardiorespiratory system along with your muscles.

POINTS TO REMEMBER ABOUT YOUR ENERGY WORKOUT

- *Before embarking on your energy workout program, check with your doctor to rule out physical disorders such as thyroid malfunction that might be depleting your energy.*
- *Start your energy workout with light weights and progress slowly at first, allowing up to four weeks to toughen up for more rugged energy workouts.*
- *After four weeks, begin using the Weider Overload Principle for progressive energy gains.*
- *Work out three times each week on alternate days—either Monday, Wednesday and Friday, or Tuesday, Thursday and Saturday.*
- *For increased energy without injury, it's important to perform all your energy exercises with a controlled, steady rhythm.*
- *You must eat a well-balanced diet and get enough sleep to derive maximum benefit from your energy workouts.*

For those whose physical condition and motivation allow, additional physical activities can be added to the overall program. On the days you don't train with weights you can walk, jog, swim, ride a bike or engage in racket sports, etc. The important point to remember is: always increase the workload when possible. When you have moved up to 15 reps with a weight that previously allowed only 12 reps, increase the weight by about 10%. When you find that the eight laps you've been swimming is getting too easy, go up to 10 laps. By progressively increasing your work capacity in this manner you also up your energy levels. However, strict precaution must be exercised so that you don't overdo it by attempting too much too soon. That will only make you weak and fatigued, and discourage you from continuing with your exercise program.

If, for whatever reason, you're forced to miss a workout, make up for the lost activity in substitute fashion. If your place of work isn't in a high-crime district, you might park your car a half mile from the office and walk. You might set aside some time at lunch and perform a series of free-hand or calisthenic-type exercises.

Part and parcel of an effective energy program is proper nutrition. Without a well-balanced diet the body will not have the resources required for the creation of optimal energy. A well-balanced diet is one that supplies the body's daily requirements of protein, fats, carbohydrates, minerals, vitamins and water.

A well-rounded energy diet would include two or more servings from the Four Basic Food Groups: cereals and grains; milk and dairy products; fruits and vegetables; meats, fish and poultry. Bear in mind that there is no one food substance or nutritional element that will provide you super energy. It is only by exercising regularly, eating properly, getting enough rest and avoiding energy "leaks" that you'll achieve optimal energy.

It's also important that your body's muscle-to-fat ratio is what it should be. There is no greater scourge to energy production than obesity. Obesity—the result of eating more calories than you expend as energy—does not happen overnight. Fat accumulates furtively, one morsel of food at a time. A calorie-laden meal or snack before bed on a regular basis represents trouble. Consuming only 100 calories a day more than the body's maintenance needs adds up to about 10 pounds of fat gained in a year. A recent study of physical activity at the University of Pennsylvania showed that physical activity plays a significant role in weight control. The study showed that oftentimes obese people actually ate *less* than thinner people. The reason they were fatter is that they weren't exercising as much.

LOOKING FOR ENERGY "LEAKS"

It's possible to train regularly and eat properly, yet still suffer an inexplicable lack of drive and energy. This is usually the result of any of a number of energy "leaks" which act insidiously to rob you of precious energy. Energy "leaks" are often subtle and hard to detect unless you know what to look for. The following are some of the more common causes of energy drain:

1. There is a mental and emotional side to low energy. Boredom can rob you of energy. When you don't take the time and effort to continually cultivate new and demanding interests, life begins to lose its luster. A continual flow of "newness" into your life acts as a kind of "magic" which increases your energy and enthusiasm without your even trying.

Unresolved conflicts and negative emotions can dam up our energies. When the subconscious mind is preoccupied with the resolution of long-standing conflicts, it's not free to perceive and experience life afresh each and every moment. If you're having trouble resolving a conflict, see a trained professional.

2. Lack of sleep will also drain you of energy. The value of regular sleep in giving us greater energy and a longer life span has even been accepted by life insurance companies.

A light nap after lunch is a great restorer of energy, as Winston Churchill proved. Studies at Stephens College, Missouri, showed that when students slept for an hour after lunch their scholastic performance was better than when they used the time for studying.

The proper amount of sleep for your individual temperament is important to build your energy bank to the highest possible level. If you seem to require nine hours, don't let anyone talk you out of it. Others might get by with six or seven hours, which is fine, but if you require more, by all means get it.

3. Stress—if it's nonproductive—can drain a person's energy reserve. Dr. Allan Hobson of the University of Massachusetts Mental Health Center says, "Stress attacks people who are expending energy and not getting anywhere."

In many cases our anxieties and worries are magnified by the buildup of tension. Physical exercise aids in skimming off the tensions and frustrations, thus robbing neurosis of its fuel.

4. Alcohol and smoking are two habits that are sure to put a damper on your energy. Think of the hours on your derriere, immobile, drinking; the hours spent recuperating from the effects of alcohol; and the effects on your physical condition year after year. Alcohol has never created energy; it burns it up.

Smoking is just about as bad as alcohol in sabotaging your energy. Dr. Jean Mayer, Harvard nutritionist, states that heavy cigarette smoking is more injurious to health than obesity. "Depending on one's age," he says, "a pack of cigarettes a day may have the same deleterious effect as 50 to 100 pounds of excess weight."

5. Don't think you can beat an energy deficiency with pep pills. That's akin to whipping a tired horse. These pills never attack or resolve the underlying cause of tiredness. They only present the danger of overwork through artificial stimulation, thus compounding your problem. Moreover, pep pills can be addictive. Stay away from them.

If the individual hopes to fulfill his potential, he must have an adequate supply of the fuel required to pursue his goals. Again, there is nothing magical or mystical about the source of

ENERGY: KEEP YOURS AT MUSCLE-BUILDING LEVELS 73

energy. The cause-and-effect relationship between sound living principles and a happy, energetic life has been espoused by the Weider organization for decades. Joe Weider and his team of champions worldwide are living proof that the principles explained here invariably work for everyone willing to put forth the effort and incorporate them into his or her lifestyle. So join the Weider team, get energized and become a superachiever!

YOUR ENERGY WORKOUT EXERCISES

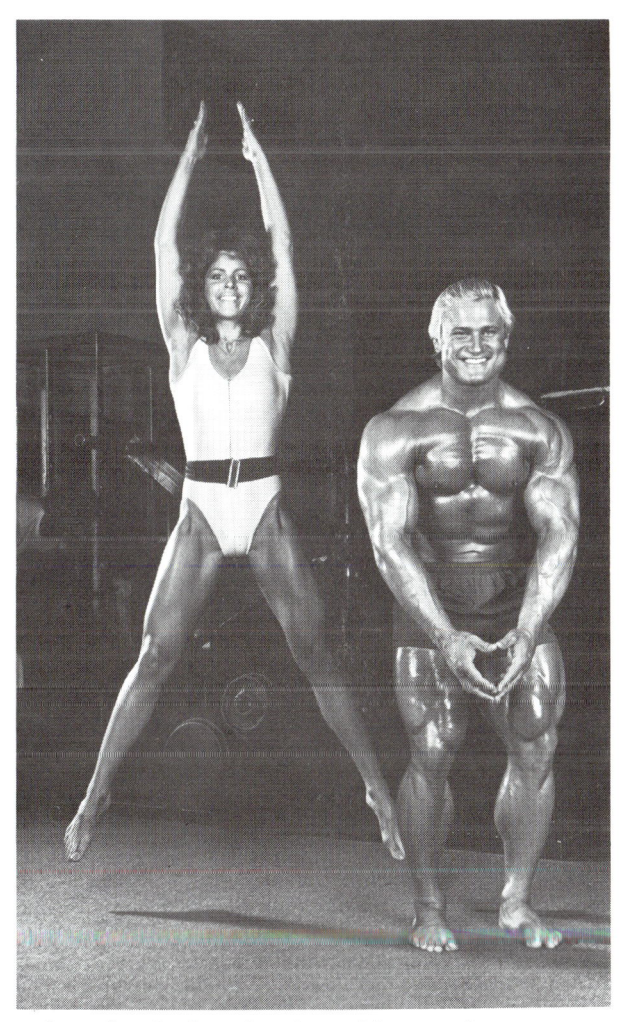

Jumping Jacks—Starting with your feet together and hands at your sides, jump at least six inches in the air and thrust your legs sideways while simultaneously clapping your hands overhead; then immediately return to the starting position, all in one movement. Jumping Jacks are great for an overall body warm-up and for increasing the circulation.

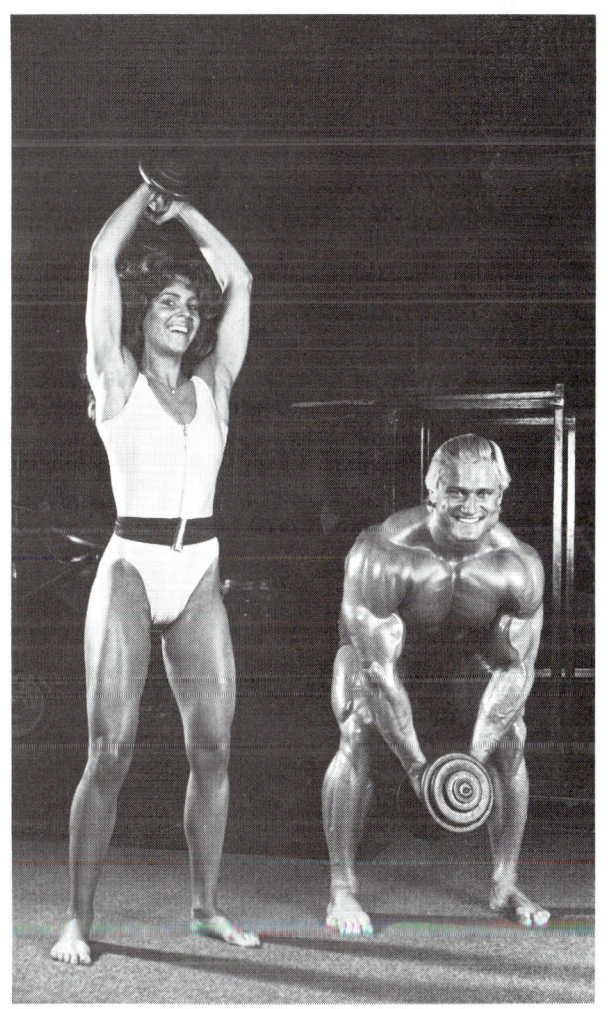

Dumbbell Swings—With your feet slightly more than shoulder width apart, hold a dumbbell with both hands between your legs. With a sudden, controlled thrust, bring the dumbbell overhead and stand straight up. Great for toning all the muscles on the back of the body.

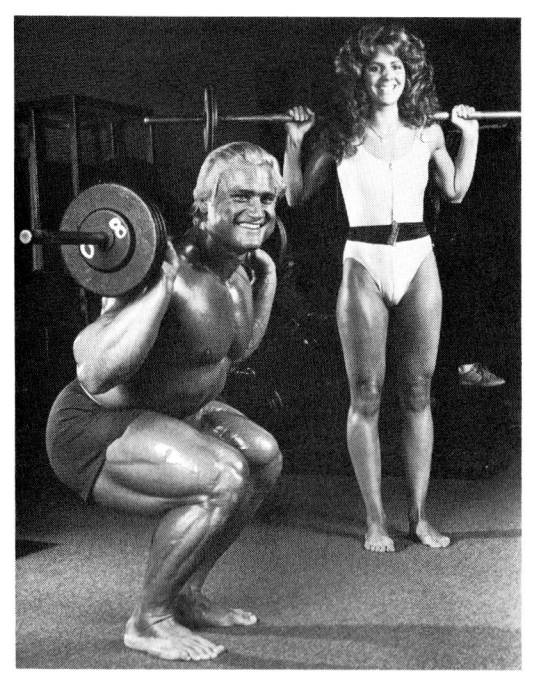

Squats—While holding a barbell across your shoulders and with your head up and back straight, bend your knees until your thighs are parallel with the floor, then stand back up. Squats are the best exercise for the front of the thighs and are great for increasing your energy.

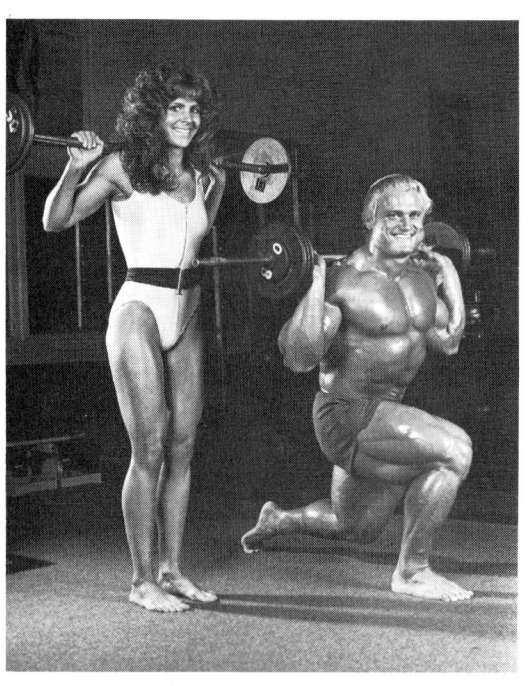

Lunges—Holding a barbell across your shoulders, lunge forward with your left leg until your right leg is straight behind you. Step back to the starting position immediately and repeat with the opposite leg. Lunges firm the buttocks and the area around the knees.

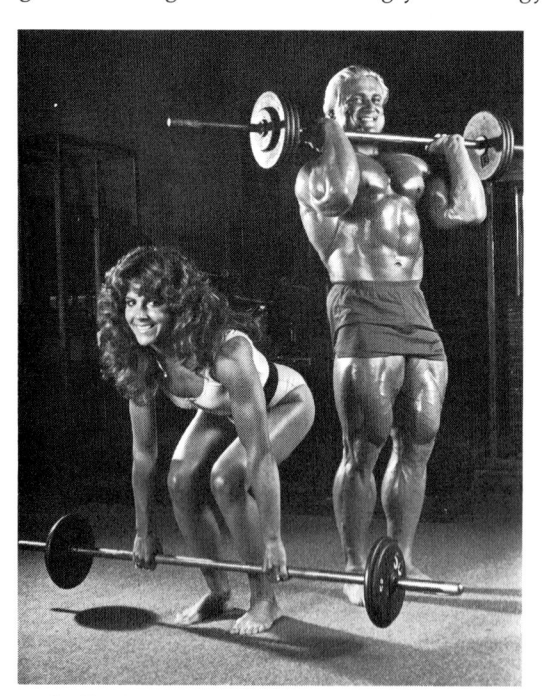

Barbell Cleans—With your back flat and your head up, grab the bar evenly with a shoulder-width grip. Keeping your back flat and head up, in one motion bring the barbell up to your shoulders and lower it. Cleans work the upper back muscles and are a great body conditioner.

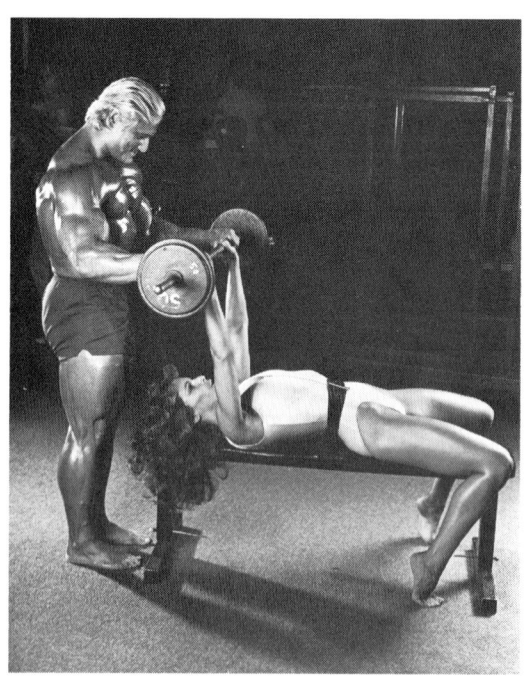

Bench Press—Using a shoulder-width grip, remove the bar from the rack. Lower the barbell under control to midchest, pause momentarily, then press back to the top under control. Great for the chest, shoulders and back of the arms.

ENERGY: KEEP YOURS AT MUSCLE-BUILDING LEVELS 75

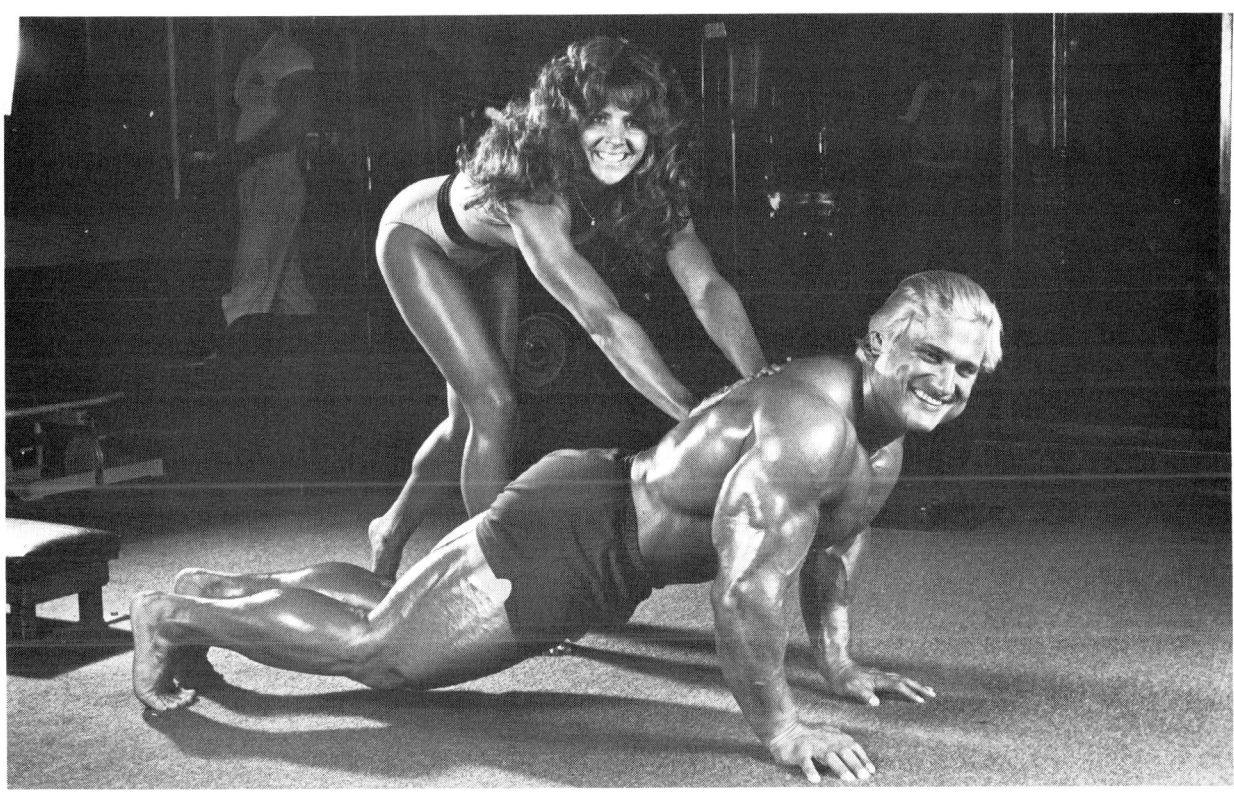

Push-Ups—Support yourself parallel to the floor with your hands directly under your thorax. Keeping your back straight, without sagging, lower yourself until just your ribcage touches the floor, then push yourself back to the top. Push-Ups are fabulous for toning the chest muscles and the back of the arms.

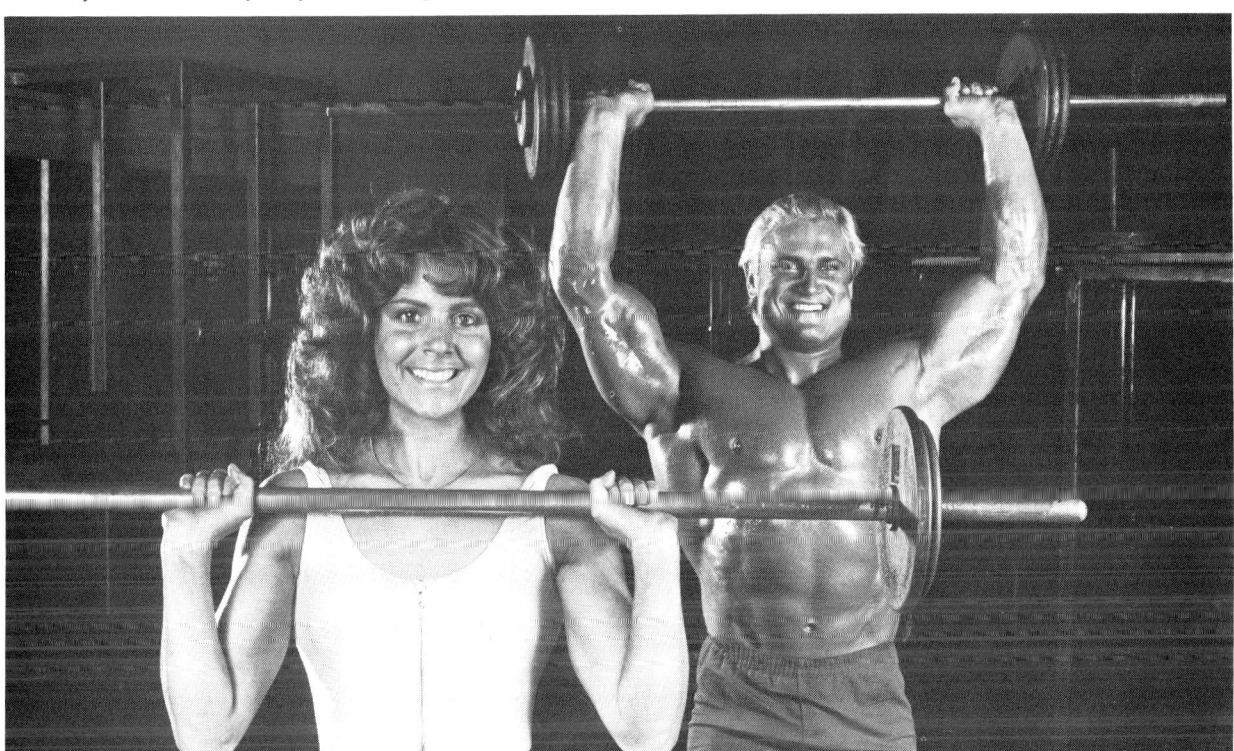

Barbell Press—Keeping the back and knees straight, press the bar overhead using a shoulder-width grip, then lower under control. Primarily a shoulder toner.

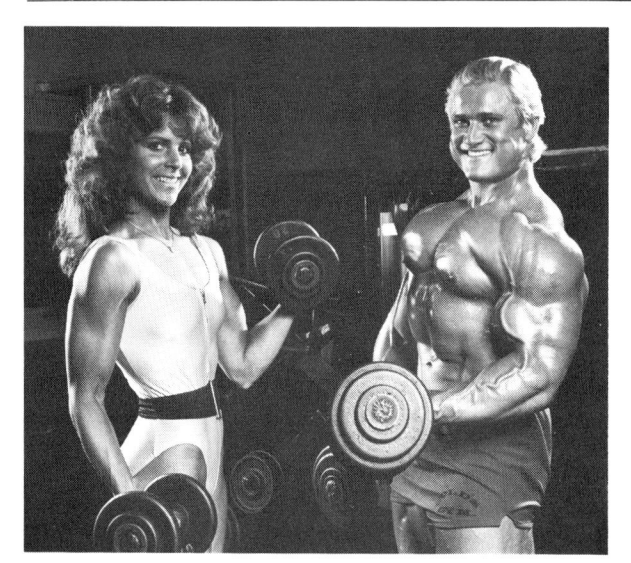

Dumbbell Curls—*Slowly curl the dumbbells (either together or alternately) to the chest, pause, then lower under control. Builds biceps and grip.*

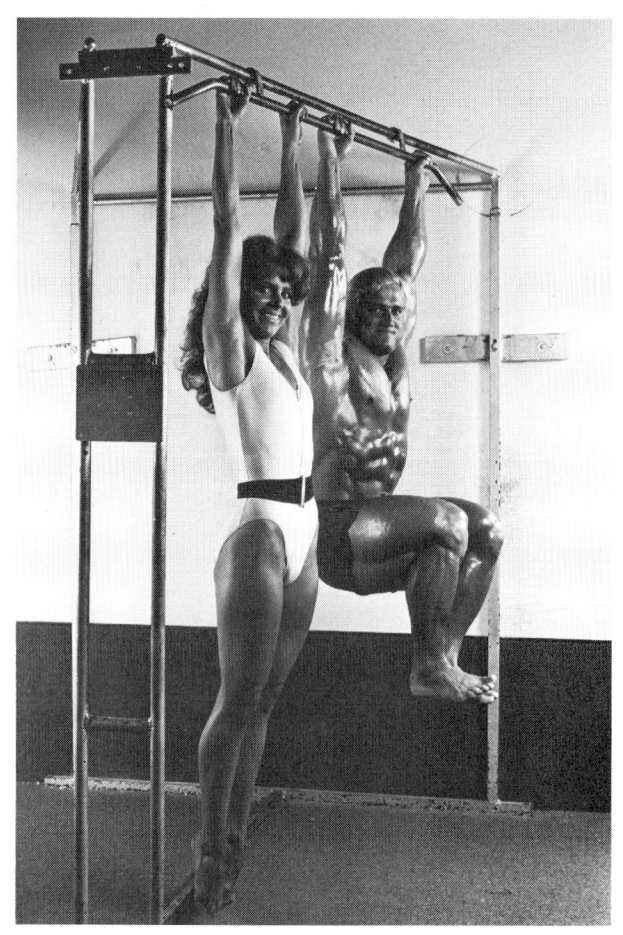

Leg Raises from chinning bar—*While hanging from a chinning bar and with your knees slightly bent, raise your legs until your thighs touch your torso, then lower your legs. Tightens up the entire midsection.*

You Can Create a World-Class Waist

by Candy Csencsits, as told to Bill Reynolds

I'd never seen anything like Auby Paulik's crisply defined abdominal formation, and I almost gasped in astonishment as I watched her pose at the 1980 Miss Olympia. Even though my own waistline was shapeless, out-of-tone and coated with a layer of fat, I vowed then, as I watched my first physique contest that evening, one day to have abs to rival Auby's. I'm not there yet, but I'm closing the gap.

That night I went home and—as late as it was—I looked through every back issue of *Muscle & Fitness* that my husband Frank had saved. From the information they contained I mapped out a plan of attack for shaping up my midsection. It worked so well and so quickly for me that I'd like to share it with you.

First of all, for complete development and maximum sharpness in the midsection, I believe that the abdominal muscles should be trained every day and from a wide variety of angles. The seven waist exercises described in this article are my favorites, but I also do many other waist movements frequently.

In the off season I do 1000 reps a day of abdominal work. Before a show I often alternate days of doing 3000 reps with days of performing only 1000. This approach has worked quite well for me.

I like to do between 200 and 400 reps of each exercise, but for the most intense training movements, like Hanging Leg Raises, Incline Leg Raises and Incline Sit-Ups, it's difficult to do more than 25–50 reps at a time.

In each workout I choose a different combination of exercises to keep my abdominal muscles off-balance and responsive to training. Any muscle group will refuse to improve if trained on the same program too long. By constantly changing my routines I am, of course, applying the Weider Muscle Confusion Training Principle. I also like to use the Weider Continuous Tension Training Principle in my ab workouts.

Ordinarily I train my major muscle groups in the morning. Then I set aside 30–60 minutes at night to concentrate strictly on training my midsection. By isolating my abdominal workout from the rest of my body like this I am using the Weider Double-Split System and Muscle Priority Training Principles. Without these principles, I couldn't have made the super-fast progress I have in shaping and defining my waistline.

For contest sharpness in the abdominal region you must follow a strict diet to allow your body to burn away fatty deposits over the muscles. Aerobic exercise also helps to burn off excess fat prior to competition.

The pre-contest diet I follow is low in fats and therefore low in calories. One gram of fat yields nine calories, vs. four calories for a gram of

77

protein or a gram of carbohydrate, so it makes sense to avoid fats like the plague when you're trying to get cut.

If you are a total beginner to bodybuilding, you should break into abdominal training gradually to avoid becoming too sore. Work your midsection only every other day for a few weeks before gradually blending into daily training. And perform only one set of a single exercise for your first couple of workouts. Then add a new set (preferably in the form of a different exercise) every second or third workout, as your abdominal muscles become more accustomed to the training.

Don't count reps. Instead, continue to do each exercise until you feel a slight burning sensation in the abdominal muscles. Even if this means halting a set after only 10 reps at first, don't worry. Your abdominals will very quickly grow accustomed to doing high reps (50 and more) each set.

In case you're confused about how to vary your workouts, here are three different beginning routines that you can use (see the photos and exercise descriptions accompanying this article for the correct way to perform each movement):

Alternative # 1
Seated Twisting
Low-Incline Sit-Ups
Knee-Ups

Alternative # 2
Low-Incline Leg Raises
Twisting Sit-Ups
Crunches

Alternative # 3
Knee-Ups
Seated Twisting
Low-Incline Sit-Ups

For the first two or three weeks, do just one set of each movement and perform only a "comfortable" number of reps.

As you progress into the intermediate level of bodybuilding training, you can probably do one set each of four or five exercises. And eventually you can do 10–15 total sets if that's what your body seems to require. This could involve **performing three sets each of five different exercises, two sets each of seven or eight movements, or one set each of 15 different exercises.**

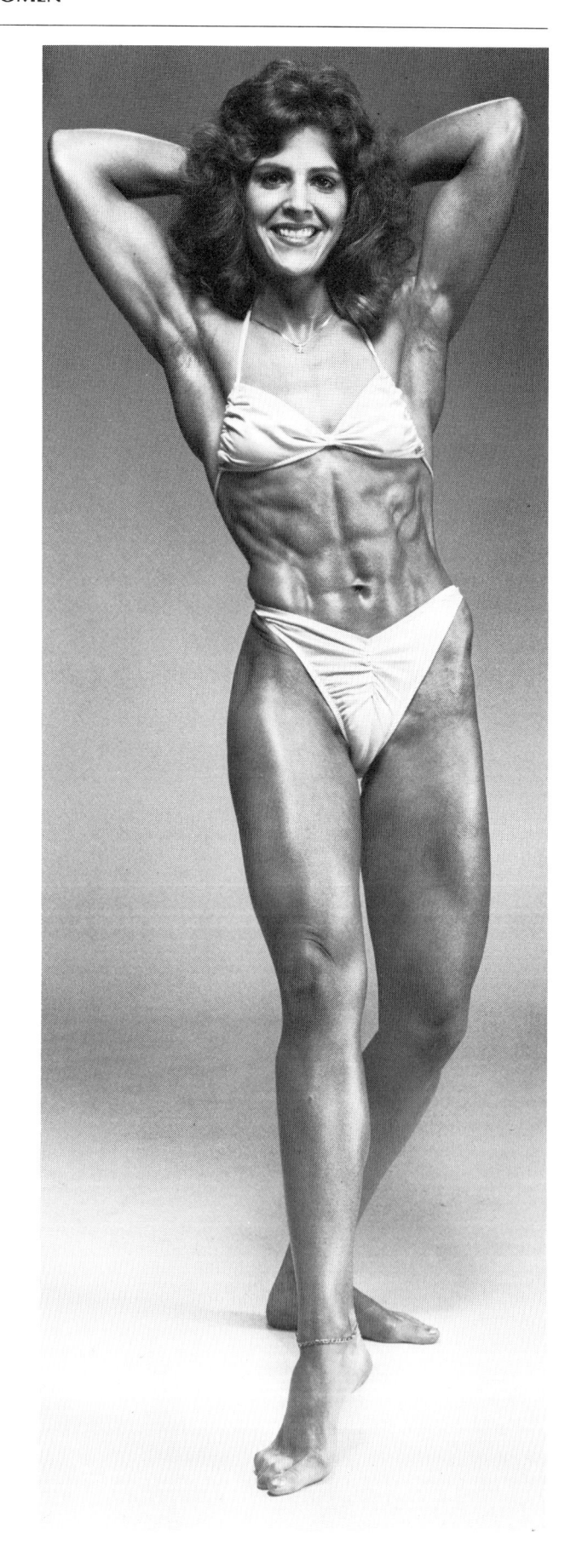

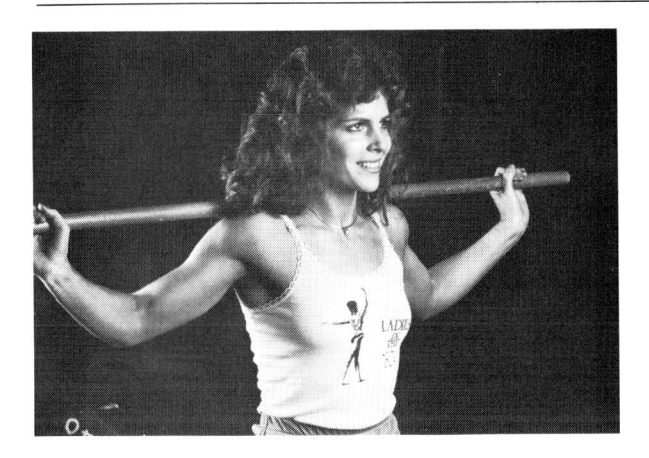

Do not feel obligated to stick to just the seven waist exercises described here. There are 20–30 more that you can use; I use them from time to time to add variety to my routine. *Muscle & Fitness* doesn't have the space to illustrate all these movements, so we're focusing on my seven favorite waist exercises.

You'll pick up new abdominal movements as you go along, either by reading *Shape* and *Muscle & Fitness,* or by watching others train. Don't be afraid to try each new movement, and if it brings results, include it regularly in your workouts.

As you proceed with your bodybuilding program, keep in mind the six keys to successful abdominal training I've named in this article:

1. Daily midsection workouts (perhaps resting on Sundays, particularly in the off-season).
2. High repetitions.
3. Use of a wide variety of exercises (this utilizes the Weider Muscle Confusion Training Principle).
4. Consistent use of the Weider Continuous Tension Training Principle.
5. Use of the Weider Muscle Priority Training Principle.
6. A low-fat/low-calorie diet.

If you faithfully follow these six maxims, you'll soon have a set of abs to be proud of!

EXERCISE DESCRIPTIONS

INCLINE SIT-UPS

1. *Emphasis*—This movement stresses the entire frontal abdominal wall, particularly the upper half of the frontal abs.
2. *Starting Position*—Lie on your back on an abdominal board set on a low incline. Your feet should be toward the upper end of the board. Hook your feet under the roller pads or strap provided to restrain them. Bend your legs at a 30-degree angle to remove potential strain from your lower back as you do the movement. Either place your hands behind your head or cross your arms over your chest during the movement.
3. *The Movement*—Slowly curl your torso up off the board by first lifting your shoulders. Then follow through by lifting your upper back, middle back and lower back from the board. Sit up until your torso is perpendicular to the floor. Return to the starting point by reversing the procedure.
4. *Training Tips*—Never jerk your torso erect by throwing your head and shoulders forward and upward. The higher you set the foot end of the abdominal board, the greater the stress as you do the Sit-Ups.

TWISTING SIT-UPS

1. *Emphasis*—Doing Twisting Sit-Ups stresses the same muscles as doing Incline Sit-Ups, but also brings the intercostal muscles strongly into play.
2. *Starting Position*—This is identical to that of Incline Sit-Ups.
3. *The Movement*—Curl your torso erect as in an Incline Sit-Up, but as you do so, smoothly twist your torso to the left so that your shoulders have moved in a quarter circle by the time you have come fully up. Lower yourself back to the starting position by reversing the procedure, and repeat the movement, twisting this time to the right. Twist alternately to the left and right with each repetition.
4. *Training Tips*—Follow the tips given for Incline Sit-Ups.

INCLINE LEG RAISES

1. *Emphasis*—This movement stresses the entire frontal abdominal wall, particularly the lower half of the frontal abs.
2. *Starting Position*—Lie on your back on an abdominal board set on a low incline. Your head should be toward the elevated end of the board. Grasp the roller pads or strap with your hands to hold your torso on the board during the movement. Bend your legs at a 30-degree angle to prevent strain on your lower back. Press your legs together while doing the movement.
3. *The Movement*—From the starting position, slowly raise your legs upward so your feet travel

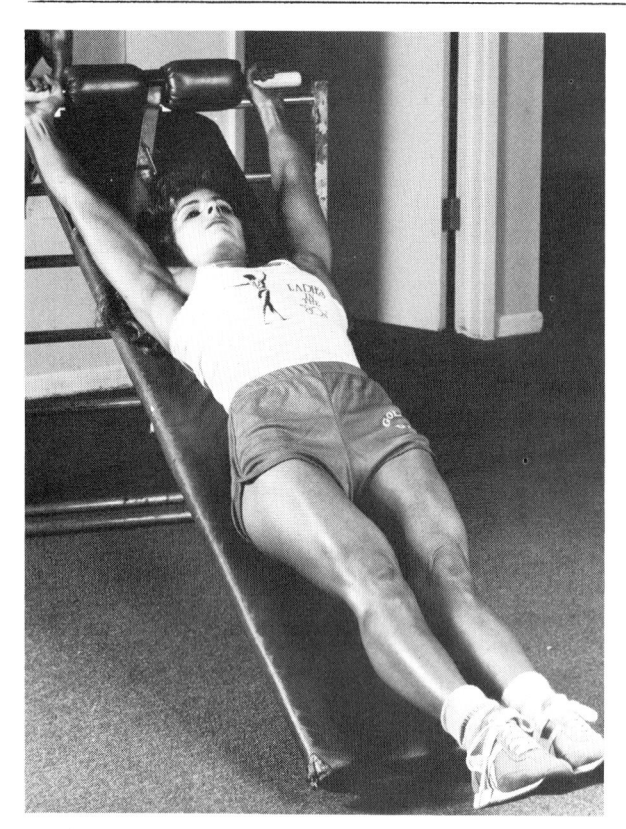

Starting position for Incline Leg Raises.

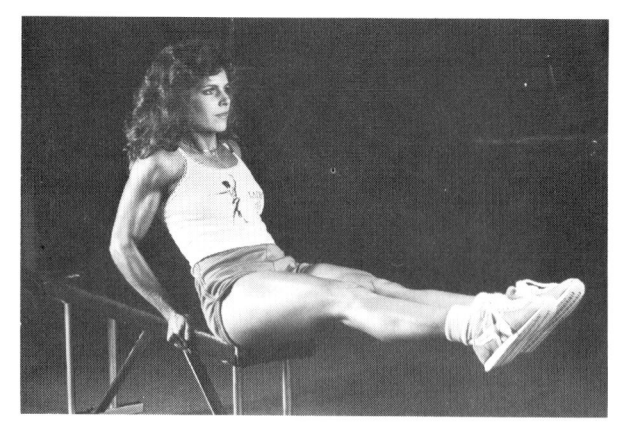

Knee-Ups—start, above; finish, below.

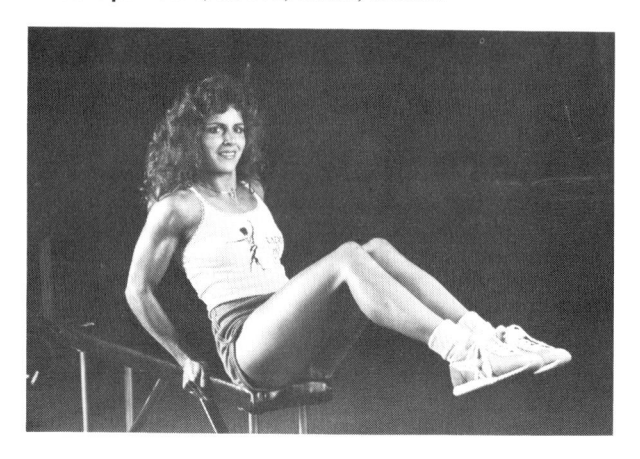

in a quarter circle from the bench to a position directly above your hips. Lower your feet to the starting point and repeat the movement for the required number of reps.

4. *Training Tips*—The higher the head end of the abdominal board, the greater the stress on your abdominals. To add Continuous Tension to the movement, bring your feet down until they don't quite touch the board, and then begin to raise them again.

KNEE-UPS

1. *Emphasis*—This movement stresses the same muscles as Incline Sit-Ups, but not as intensely.
2. *Starting Position*—Sit at the end of a flat exercise bench or on a chair. Your buttocks must be right at the end of the bench. Lean back until your torso is at a 45-degree angle with the floor. Hold onto the bench or chair to keep your torso at this angle during the exercise. Extend your legs out in front of you in such a position that they make one even line with your torso, so your body is entirely straight. At this point your feet should be just above the floor.
3. *The Movement*—Keeping your legs either pressed together or fairly close together, slowly pull your knees up to your chest, bending your legs fully as you do so. Hold the top position for a moment and then reverse the procedure to lower your legs back to the starting position.
4. *Training Tip*—To increase the intensity of this movement, you can wear iron boots.

CRUNCHES

1. *Emphasis*—This movement stresses the entire frontal abdominal wall.
2. *Starting Position*—There are several variations. In the basic position, you lie on your back and drape your lower legs over a flat exercise bench, with knees bent so your thighs are perpendicular to the floor. Then you place your hands behind your head. Alternatively, you can assume this position with your legs in the air without a bench to support them. You can also do the movement with your legs running up a wall and your buttocks against the wall as you lie on the floor, or you can assume the basic starting position with your feet or toes placed against the wall. Instead of holding your hands behind your head, you can cross your arms over your chest.

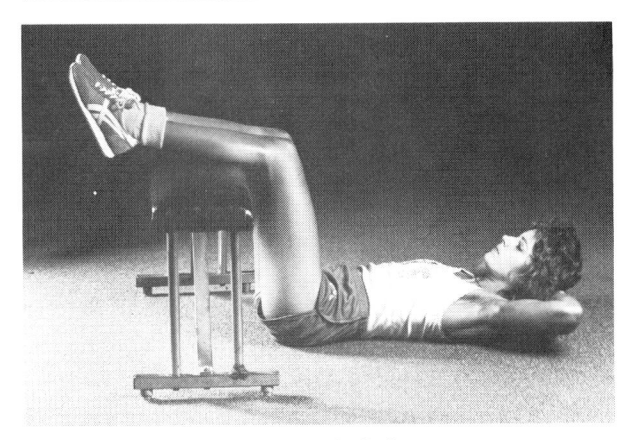

Crunches—start, above; finish, below.

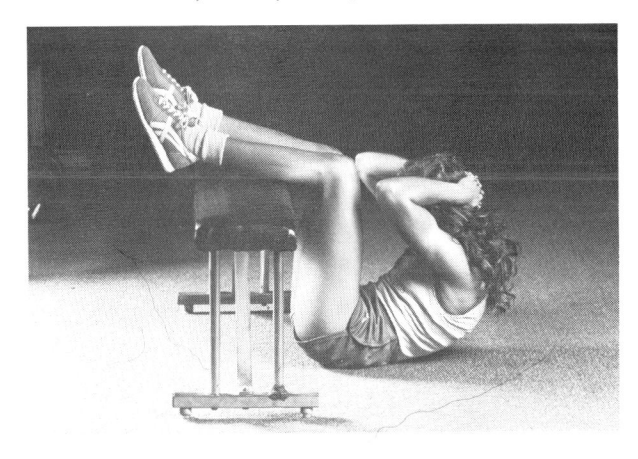

3. *The Movement*—You must do four things simultaneously: 1) Raise your shoulders and upper back up off the floor; 2) Raise your hips from the floor; 3) Blow out all of the air in your lungs as forcibly as possible; 4) Try to force your shoulders toward your hips, "shortening" your torso. Hold the top position momentarily and then relax your abdominal muscles to lower yourself back to the starting position. Repeat the movement for the required number of repetitions.

4. *Training Tip*—As with Twisting Sit-Ups, you can stress the intercostal muscles if you twist your shoulders a little to each side as you do the movement.

HANGING LEG RAISES

1. *Emphasis*—This exercise stresses all of the muscles of the frontal abdominal wall, particularly the lower abdominal muscles.

2. *Starting Position*—Grasp a chinning bar with a shoulder-width grip and hang. You may wish to wear gloves to protect your hands as you grip the bar.

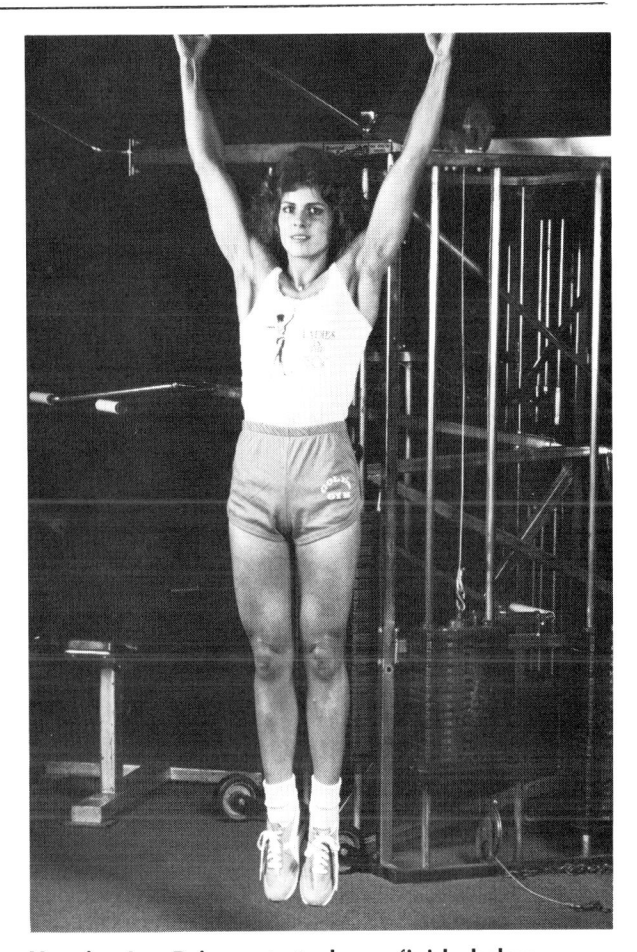

Hanging Leg Raises—start, above; finish, below.

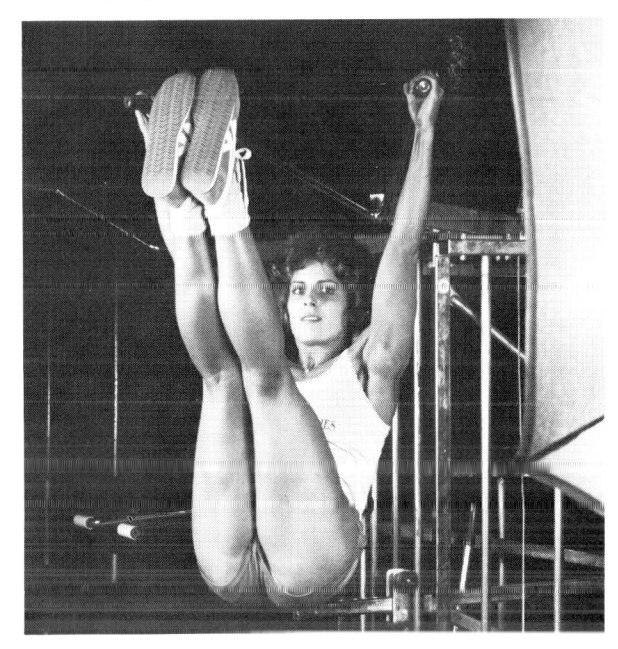

3. *The Movement*—There are two basic approaches. In the easier version, you pull your knees upward while bending your legs, until your knees either touch your chest or come very

close. This movement is very similar to that done in Knee-Ups. In the more difficult version of Hanging Leg Raises, you bend your legs about 15 degrees during the movement and raise your feet in quarter circles until they are above a line drawn through your hips and parallel to the floor, then lower to the starting position.

4. *Training Tips*—You might begin to swing a little from the bar as you do these. If so, simply have a training partner hold your hips in position by grasping the sides of your waist or hips. By twisting slightly to each side, you can work the intercostal muscles as you do the movement.

SEATED TWISTING

1. *Emphasis*—This movement tones and firms the muscles at the sides of your waist. It also loosens up your lower back.

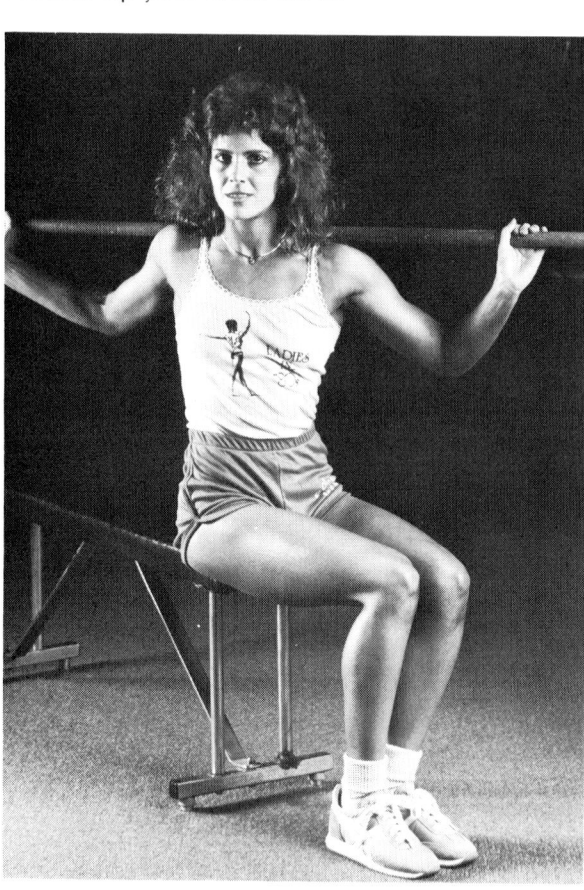

2. *Starting Position*—Sit astride a flat exercise bench and either place your feet flat on the floor or wrap your legs around the upright legs of the bench. This second position is better because it more effectively keeps your hips from moving. Place a broomstick or an unloaded barbell behind your neck and either wrap your arms around it or grasp the ends.

3. *The Movement*—From this basic starting position, twist your shoulders as far to the left as you can. Then immediately and rather quickly twist as far as you can to the right. Twist rhythmically from side to side for the desired number of repetitions.

4. *Training Tip*—Never add weight to this movement! Doing so could enlarge the external oblique muscles at the sides of your waist, making your waistline look wider. And that's something you don't want.☐

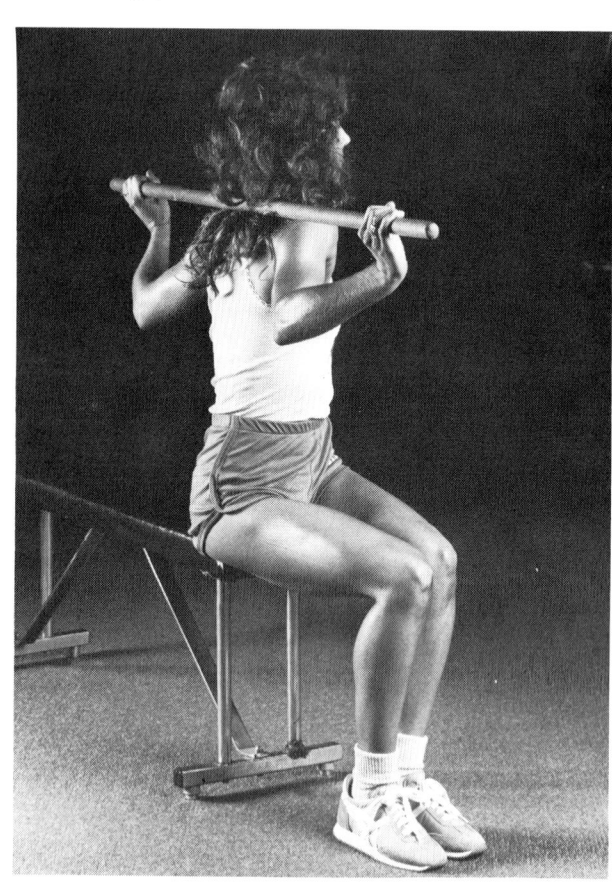

Seated Twisting.

Shaping the Chest—Kike Elomaa Style

by Rick Wayne

Recently, while Britain teetered on the brink of civil war and California's farmers girded their loins to meet the threat of the medfly, while Poland's Solidarity and the guerillas of El Salvador occupied the American consciousness, something equally revolutionary, a phenomenon no less, was developing in Europe. Unreported by the world press, it had begun with the successful participation of a young Finnish nurse named Kike Elomaa in the hotly contested 1981 European Bodybuilding Championships in London. A blonde Nefertiti, Kike (key-key) had then gone on to dominate the female section of the IFBB's World Games competition in San Jose, California, a few weeks later. With barely three years of bodybuilding behind her, Kike suddenly found herself the center of attraction. Strangers stopped to compliment her on the streets of Turku, her hometown in Finland. Collectors yearned for her autograph. Some of her country's top fashion houses courted her. She signed lucrative contracts with two of Finland's leading sportswear manufacturers. The Finns had found themselves a new star, but nobody guessed what was still to come.

Late August Kike returned to the United States to take on the world's leading female bodybuilders in the year's Miss Olympia. Among the contenders were the delicious Rachel McLish, a favorite with American fans and judges, and the incredible Laura Combes.

By her own account, Kike was "not quite as fantastic" as she had planned to be for the big contest. No matter. From the moment she appeared at the Philadelphia Sheraton, where the event was staged, all eyes were glued to her. Even in full street attire, Kike was a joy to behold. She walked with a majestic gait in her knee-high boots, and rewarded admirers with a warm smile and a look in her big, blue eyes that could defrost Oscar State. Long before the contest actually began, the name you heard most was Kike Elomaa. Her husband and trainer, Kimmo, beamed.

After Kike had made the Olympia her third victory in a row, here is what Sheila Herman, a judge and reporter for *Muscle & Fitness*, had to say: "It was close   Kike led from the start . . . Kike was as close as anyone came to perfection. She is extremely charismatic, carries herself like a champion. . . ."

And the audience agreed, a phenomenon in itself these days when practically every contest result is greeted with boos from the partisan fans.

The Finnish press could hardly wait for Kike's return. As the young woman descended from her plane a score of reporters rushed her with notebooks, cameras, TV equipment and microphones. Inside the terminal it seemed half the population of Turku had come out to welcome the Elomaas home. Something incredible was going on. A raging fever had swept through Finland. The press called it Kike Emotion.

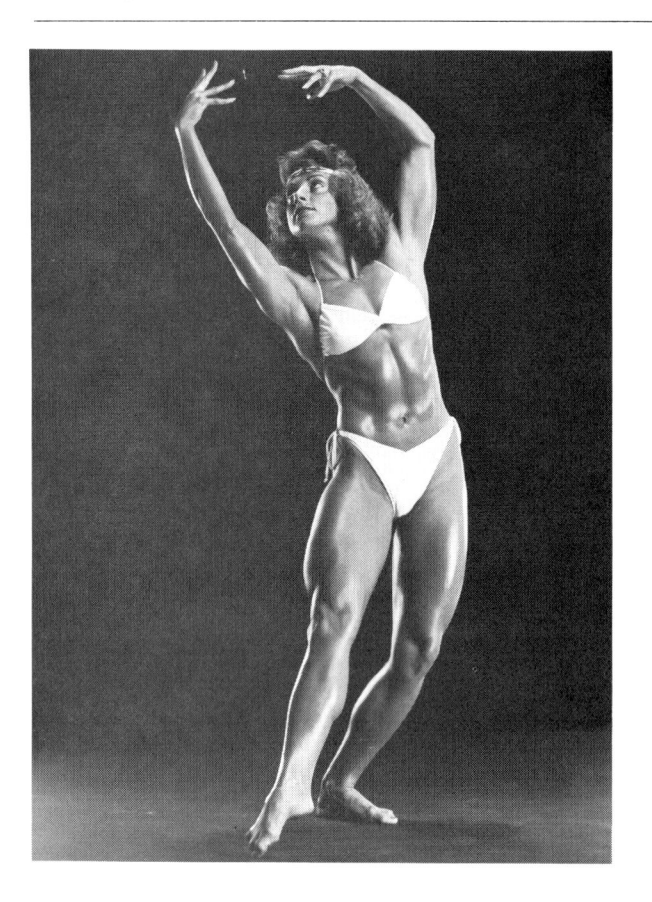

Within days Kike had signed a contract with the most prestigious recording company in Finland. She recorded two original tunes by her country's leading songwriter. Later she signed with a jeans manufacturer and broke into TV with her own bodybuilding show.

Today the Kike fever is hotter than ever. Kike's services as a guest artist on European television are in great demand, and hardly a week goes by without three or four offers from bodybuilding entrepreneurs reaching the Elomaas. Kike and Kimmo travel extensively, which is hell, considering they also own six gymnasiums that they must look after.

It's hardly surprising that in Finland, female bodybuilding has eclipsed the popularity of its older brother. With Kike leading the girls, Jorma Raty and his boys certainly have a difficult time keeping up. Recently, Kike Elomaa was voted her country's most popular woman, a title that until

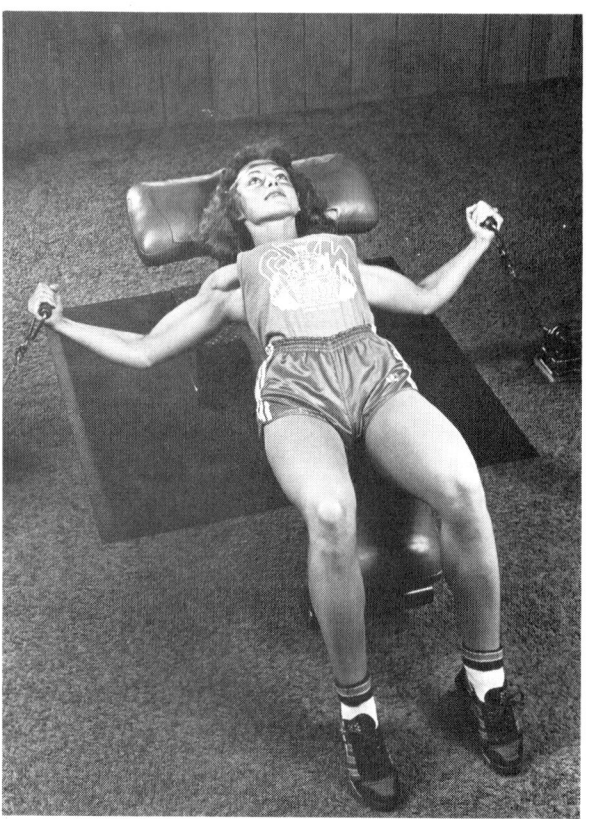

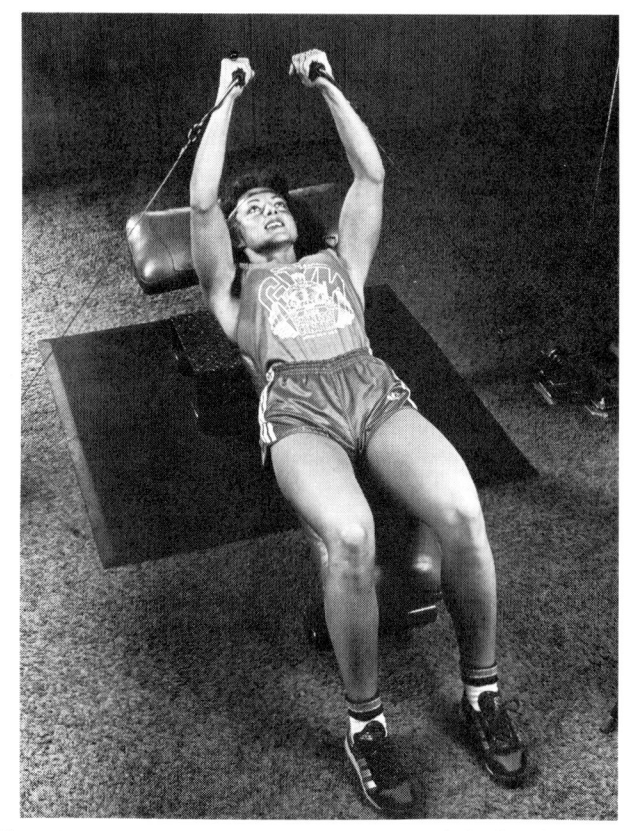

Incline Cable Flyes stress the upper pectorals with an excellent degree of continuous tension. Start, left; finish, right. Note how low Kike brings her elbows at the start to stretch her pectorals.

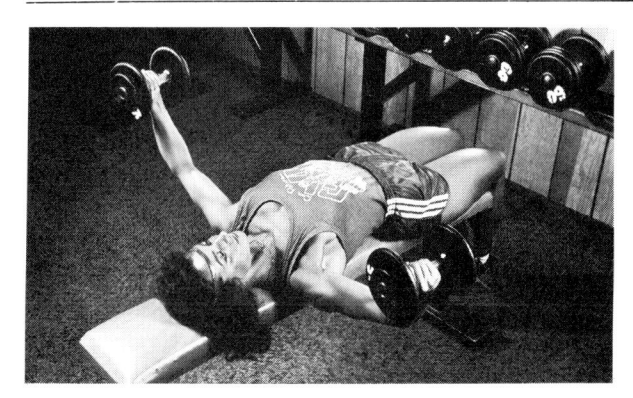

Dumbbell Flyes done on a slight decline build up and shape the lower pectorals, resulting in a full and powerful appearance for the entire chest complex.

recently belonged to the wife of the Finnish president.

Early this year Kike visited Southern California with her husband, "to get away from the snow and to discover for ourselves some of the techniques that we read about in *Muscle & Fitness* each month."

It was pleasant to note that with her new fame Kike remains the same unassuming young woman I met in London, when the Kike Emotion first surfaced. Her English had improved, even though she often asked me, "What kind of type is this thing?"

She enjoys training to a degree that must be seen to be believed. And there is the secret of her bodybuilding success. Kike actually looks forward to her training sessions. She particularly liked to work out at the Don Peters' Fitness Center in Reseda, California, mainly because she loves training with free weights. She visited other Los Angeles gyms and had good things to say about both Gold's and World, but found others "too full of machines."

Training with Kike is like taking a workout with Arnold Schwarzenegger. She has the uncanny ability to shut out everything around her as she performs a set. She uses maximum poundages, constantly strives to work with heavier weights—but not once at the expense of style. I have never known a female bodybuilder who can pump up as quickly as Kike, something which speaks volumes for her training style.

She always makes a point of thoroughly warming up her whole body before each training session. For 15 minutes or so she does stretches, toe touches and twists, not unlike a ballet dancer preparing for a workout.

She begins her chest program with Cable Flyes on an incline bench. She starts the movement

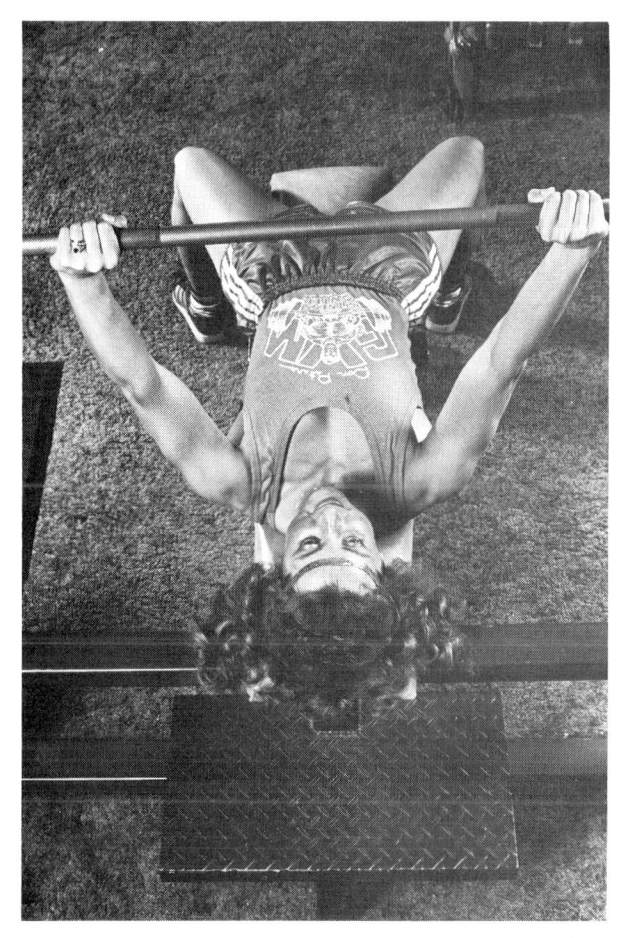

Both the Bench Press (above) and **Incline Press** (below) are essential for building chest mass and power. Even with the heaviest training poundages, Kike is careful to use very full and strict movements.

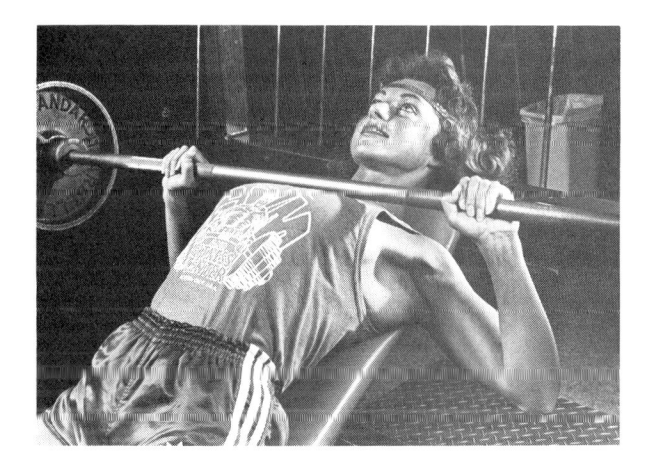

with the cable handles held at arms' length over her chest. From this point the weights are slowly lowered as far down as possible, elbows slightly bent. When her hands have reached their lowest point Kike immediately returns to the starting position. Now she relaxes for a count of two before doing the second repetition. She does a

86 BODYBUILDING AND CONDITIONING FOR WOMEN

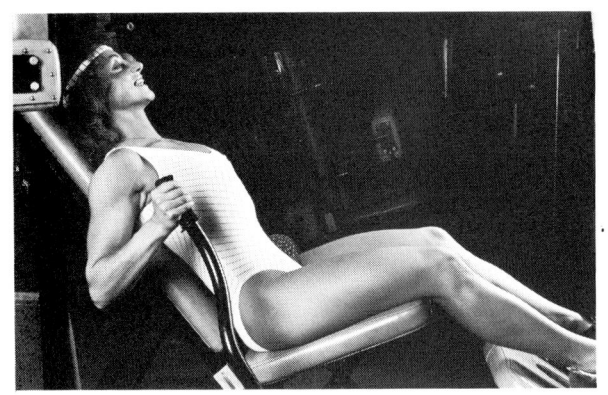

Although Kike prefers using free weights, she can perform flyes and presses on Nautilus machines for a change of pace. Nautilus Press—start, above left; finish, above right; Nautilus Flyes—start, below left; finish, below right.

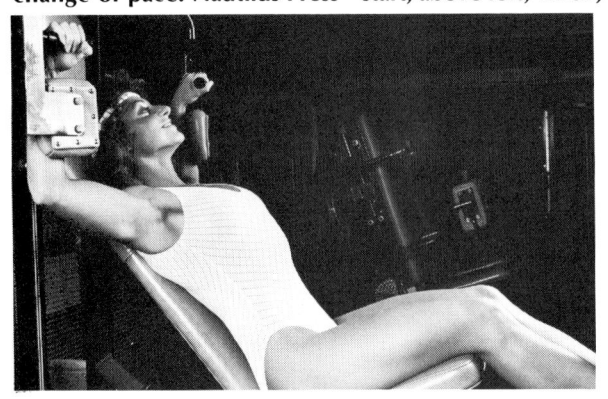

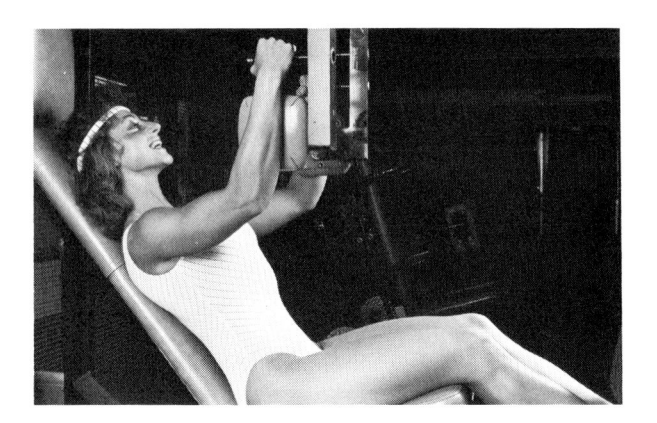

minimum of six reps and a maximum of 10. With each succeeding set she adds weight to the machine. The style never varies. Slow and concentrated. One added tip: Kike makes a point of touching the handles and keeping them together before lowering her arms. At the top position, her hands are directly over her chin, not over her chest.

She does four sets of Flyes before moving to Barbell Pullovers. She says the movement affects her rib cage, upper pecs and serratus muscles. While lying on a flat bench, she holds a light barbell at arms' length over her chest, breathes in while lowering the bar to the back of her head. She exhales as she returns to the starting position. The weight used is particularly light, so as not to interfere with the stretching of her rib cage. The hand spacing shouldn't be more than shoulder width.

Until recently Kike followed her Pullovers with Barbell Bench Presses. These days, however, she does Incline Presses with either a barbell or dumbbells.

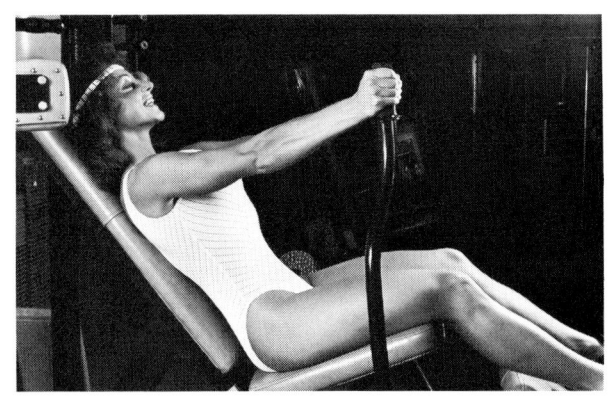

"I think there's more to be gained from Inclines," she says, "especially if the elbows are held way back and the bar is brought down to a point just below the neck."

She does two sets of Barbell Inclines, using weights heavy enough to tax her after six reps, then moves on to Dumbbell Inclines. Here she does three sets of 10 reps.

"Sometimes I will do four straight sets of either Barbell or Dumbbell Presses," says Kike, "for no particular reason except maybe variety. But I have to say I consider Barbell Inclines good for building mass and power in the upper pecs and shoulders. The dumbbell version is best for really stretching the whole upper chest."

So why not the Flat Bench Press? "It's wonderful for showing how strong you are," says Kike in an accent that was never meant for the gym. "But I don't think the Bench Press is as good a pec developer as Flyes. It works best for the triceps and deltoids."

Immediately following her chest session, Kike trains her back.□

"Look at These Shoulders"

by Dr. Lynne Pirie, D.O.

There is an old saying that says horses sweat, men perspire and women merely glow when they exercise heavily. Well, believe me, I perspire plenty when I train my shoulders. In fact, hard training is the primary reason they have developed so dramatically over the past few months.

I've had considerable education in anatomy and kinesiology. My studies in these areas have greatly aided in developing each muscle group of my body. After I explain the anatomy (structure) and kinesiology (function) of your deltoids, I am confident that you will be better able to build both mass and muscle density in your shoulders.

In simplest terms, your deltoid is a caplike muscle mass covering the top part of your upper arm bone and the point of your shoulder. The muscle originates in several places around the point of the shoulder and attaches to the outside of the upper arm bone. The deltoid has three "heads" (or lobes)—the anterior (frontal), medial (side) and posterior (rear).

The anterior head of the deltoid contracts to move the upper arm bone both forward and upward. It works simultaneously with the pectorals and triceps when doing Bench Presses at all angles with either a barbell or two dumbbells. The same is true when performing Parallel Bar Dips. Thus, when you train your chest, you usually strongly stimulate the frontal lobes of your deltoids.

All forms of Overhead Pressing—with a barbell, dumbbells, machine, etc.—directly work the anterior head of the deltoid muscle. So does the Front Raise, which can be done with a barbell, two dumbbells, or a single dumbbell held by both hands at once. Most commonly, Front Raises are done with two dumbbells in alternate fashion, one going upward as the other descends.

Overhead Pressing also affects the medial deltoid head to a degree, since that head contracts to move the upper arm bone out to the side. There are, however, more direct movements for the side delt. These include Side Lateral Raises with dumbbells, cables or various machines. I personally prefer to do Laterals on a Nautilus double-shoulder machine, but if you don't have such equipment available, use dumbbells and/or cables.

The posterior head of the deltoid contracts to move the upper arm backward and upward to the rear. As a result, these lobes respond fairly strongly to latissimus dorsi exercises such as Chins, Pulldowns and Bent Rows. You can more directly stress the posterior deltoid muscles, however, by doing various forms of Bent Laterals using dumbbells, cables or machines. With dumbbells, you can perform a Bent Lateral either

88 BODYBUILDING AND CONDITIONING FOR WOMEN

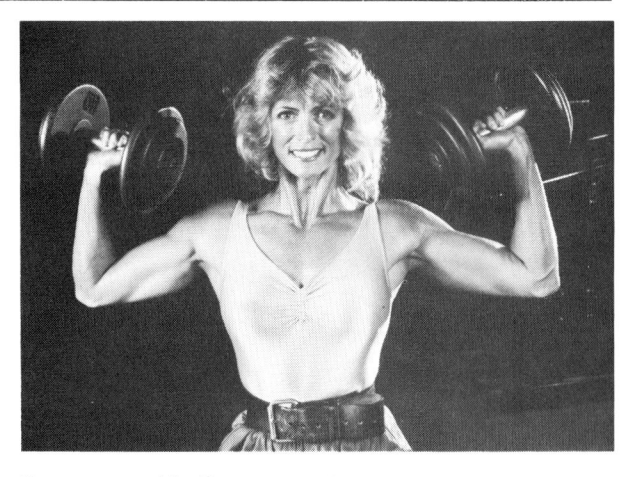

"I use Dumbbell Presses (above) once a week as an alternative to presses on a Nautilus Double-Shoulder machine. Both movements build the anteriors aspects of my shoulder muscles."

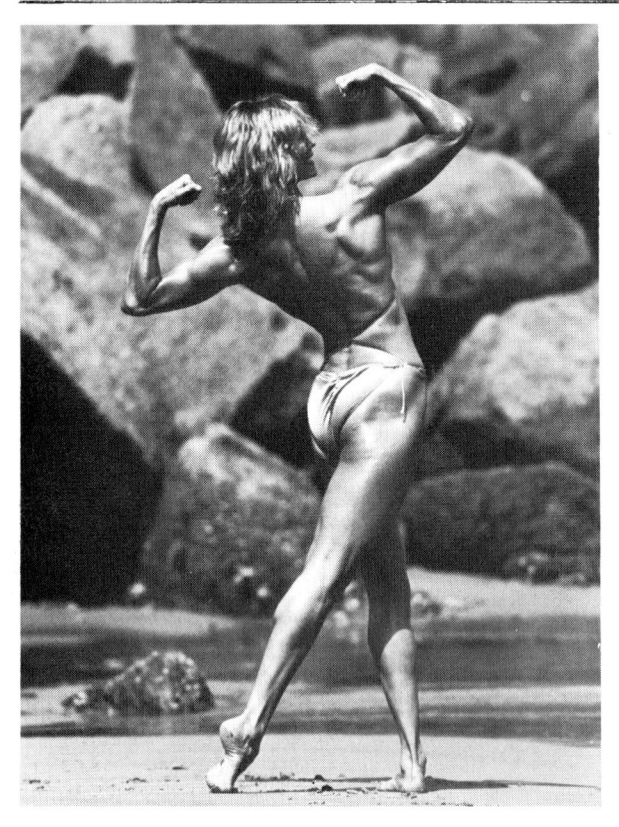

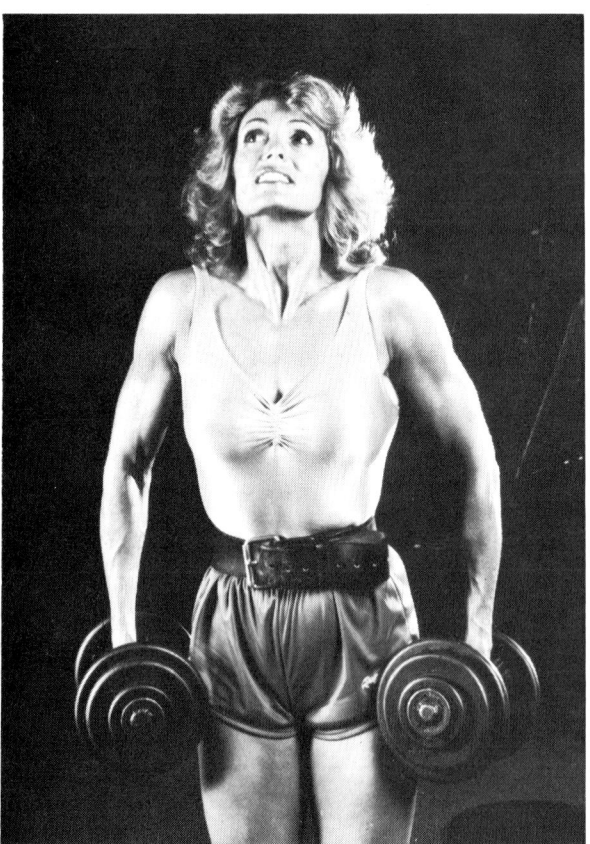

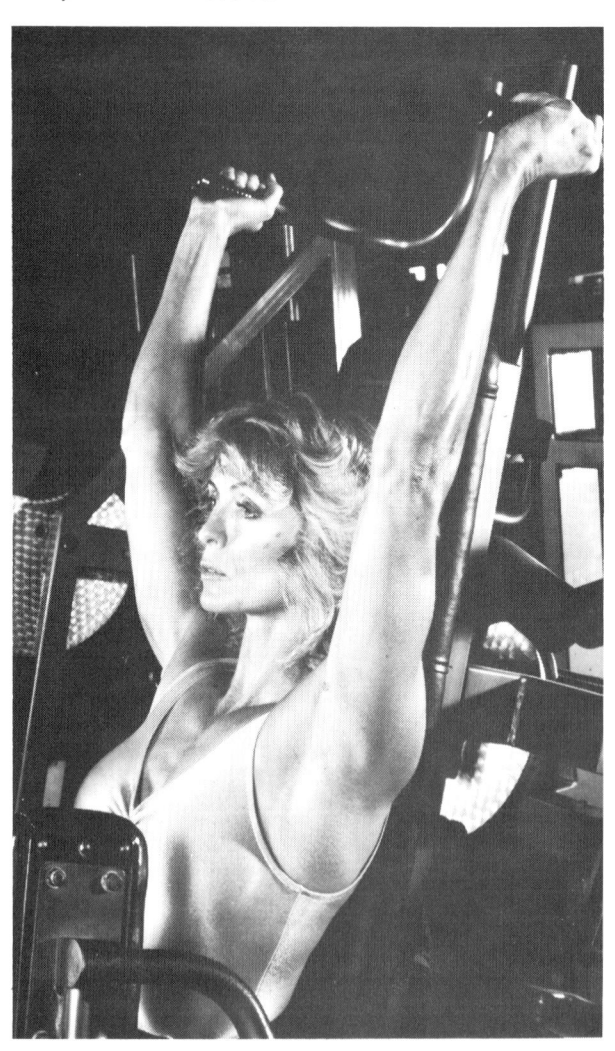

"Dumbbell Shrugs add mass to my trapezius muscles, creating a fully developed appearance to my shoulder girdle."

"LOOK AT THESE SHOULDERS" 89

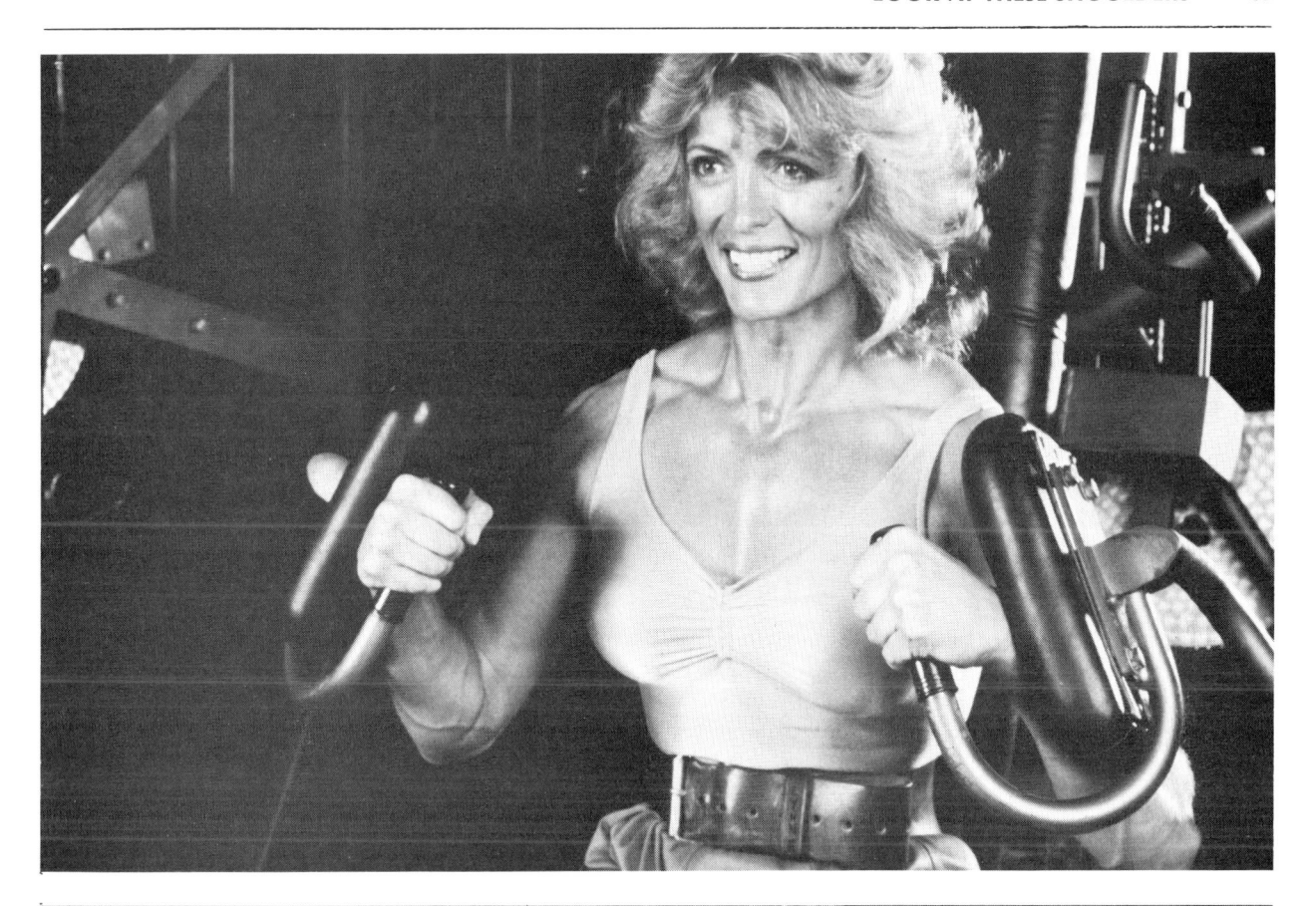

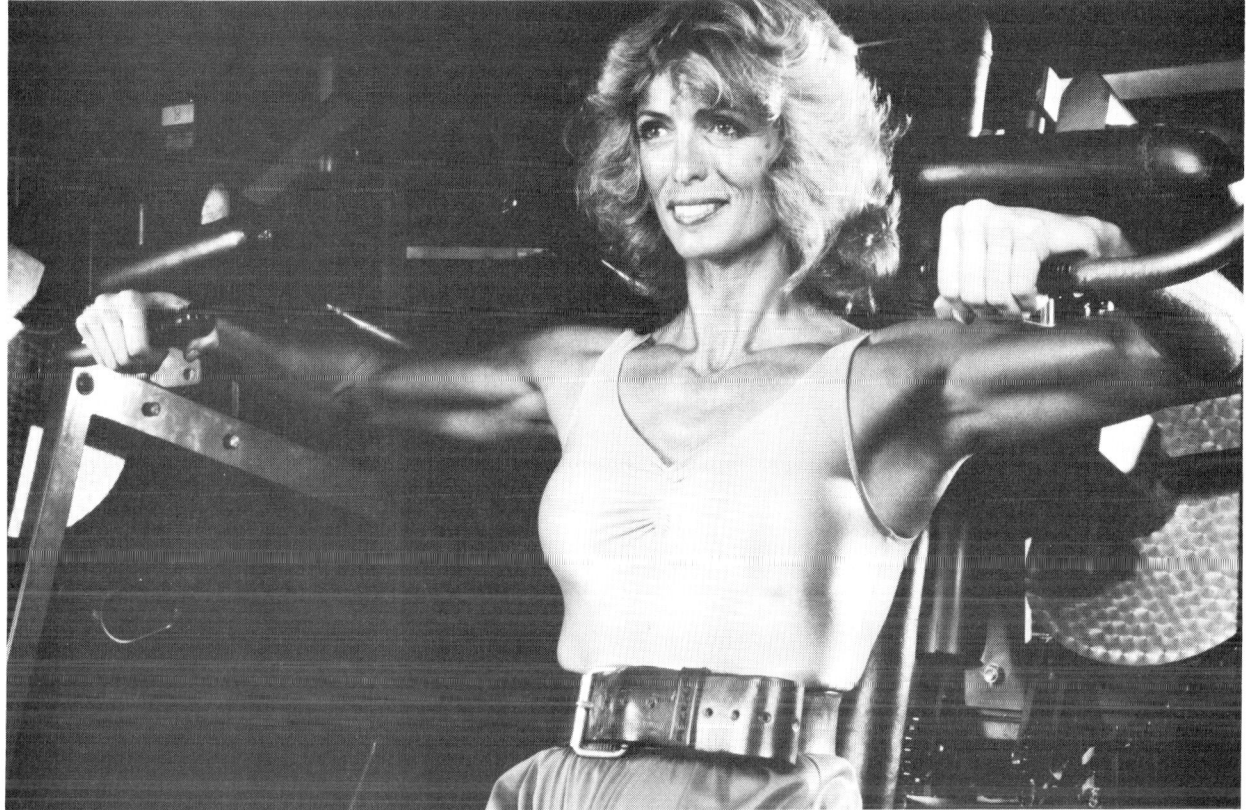

"I also use the Nautilus Double-Shoulder machine to perform Side Lateral Raises. These add mass and density to the medial heads of my deltoids."

standing or while seated at the end of a flat exercise bench.

In my training regimen, I work my deltoids on Tuesdays, Thursdays and Saturdays. I really enjoy doing my shoulder work! You could call me a sort of shoulder freak. My Tuesday and Thursday workouts are quite different from each other, while my Saturday session is a variation of my Tuesday routine. I most often work my anterior and medial deltoid heads as a unit. My rear delts are worked each training session as part of my upper back training.

I have occasionally done Dumbbell Bent Laterals, but generally I prefer a Rear-Delt Raise on a Nautilus rowing machine. According to which weekday it is, I use either the principles of forced reps and negatives, or a burnout type of down-the-rack workout. I train my rear delts with the same principles I'm using for front and side deltoids that day. You can determine my rear deltoid programs by reading the following workout description.

On Tuesdays, my workout is two-thirds completed even before I train my shoulders. By this point I've done my legs, chest and back already.

I begin by doing 10–12 good reps of Nautilus Lateral Raises with as heavy a weight as I can handle. Then my coach, Jerry Doyle, helps me force out 5–6 more reps. After a very brief rest, I do as many heavy singles as I can with about a 10-second rest-pause between efforts. Finally, I take another brief rest and do an excruciatingly difficult set of 15–20 strict-form reps with a lighter weight.

The Laterals pre-exhaust my deltoids for the Nautilus Press, which is my other Tuesday delt movement. I treat the Presses exactly like the Laterals, although I'll normally do a few more forced reps, since I exercise on a machine built specifically to let me give myself forced reps. By the time I've finished the Presses, my delts are maxed. It's a good feeling since that's what it takes to stimulate fast muscle hypertrophy.

On Thursdays I work my shoulders, although indirectly, at the beginning after which I directly stress my deltoid muscles. I first superset Pull Ups and Dips for four sets of 10–15 reps each. Then I go to Seated Dumbbell Presses supersetted with Pulldowns Behind the Neck. I do four sets of each exercise, hitting 15–20 reps on the Presses. After 10 or 12 reps, everything is forced out with Jerry's assistance. I use 40- to 45-pound dumbbells, and after 15 reps my shoulders are burning so much that it's all I can do just to hang on to the weights.

From there I move to my chest workout, starting with Incline Presses, which also strongly stress my anterior deltoids. Dumbbell Shrugs on Thursdays complete my shoulder girdle development. I do four sets with a pair of 70s, doing 15 reps, rotating my shoulders forward, and 15 reps backward. I don't use straps, however, in order to develop my grip and add to my forearm muscle mass because an orthopedic surgeon must have strong hands.

My Saturday workout is similar to Tuesday's except that I start with the heaviest possible weight and work my way down the stack. I average 6 reps with each weight and rest only 4–5 seconds between weight reductions.

Realizing that many readers won't have access to some of the equipment I use, I had John Balik photograph me doing Dumbbell Side Laterals and Seated Presses Behind the Neck. Although I have done them in the past, I don't do these exercises at present. For those without machines, they are good substitutes for Nautilus Side Laterals and Nautilus Presses.

If you don't have a coach or training partner to help you with forced reps, I'd suggest using a tri-set of Side Laterals, Presses Behind the Neck and Bent Laterals, going to failure on each exercise. This tri-set is quite good because Side Laterals pre-exhaust your delts before you do Presses. A good beginning routine consists of one or two such tri-sets. And as long as you really push each set, I don't believe that even a contest-level bodybuilder needs to do more than three of these.

The workout I follow is extremely intense, and hence result-producing. However, it could be too strenuous for less-experienced bodybuilders, leading to overtraining. Beginners certainly don't need to do forced reps, and intermediates should do only a couple of those. Make this adjustment and break in slowly to the routine and you should have no problem with my program.

You'll work like a horse and sweat like a man, but the results will be more than worth the effort. Your delts will simply explode!

"My Armful of Secrets":
Mary Roberts' Arm Training Routine

by Sheila Herman

It's hard getting the training secrets of someone who believes her secrets ought to, well, stay secret. To Mary Louise Roberts, winner of the 1981 American Women's Bodybuilding Championships (lightweight), a secret is a secret is a secret. Well, almost. She says, "Secrecy is an important part of competition. I do exercises that I name myself. It's very scientific with me and I can't explain to anyone how I do it."

It's no use trying to follow her around the gym to watch her train: she sneaks away from her regular gym eight weeks before a contest. You expect her to show off her world-class physique, but no—she's bundled up in loose fitting clothing out on the streets and she keeps her warm-up on backstage at a contest. This was one tough cookie to crack.

I had to know her secrets. So I figured: take her to a restaurant two weeks before the World Championships, ply her with salad, make her crazy with FOOD, and that will get her to talk. "Let's talk biceps, Mary Lou," I said.

"No comment," said Mary Roberts.

Well, I work for Joe Weider and I knew this wasn't going to cut it. It was drop-back-20-and-punt time. I figured, "Get what you can, Sheila." So let me tell all that is known about Mary Roberts' arm-training routine. But first, some background on Mary Lou.

Back in the dark ages of women's bodybuilding (1980), there was a contest that has never since recurred—the Robby Robinson Bodybuilding Championships. Kay Baxter won it and a striking newcomer came in second. This newcomer had trained for about three months, dieted severely for two of those months, then showed the world a type of physique previously unseen. Mary Roberts brought to the stage possibly the world's first *ripped woman bodybuilder*. At 5'3" and 95 pounds, Mary's appearance caused quite a stir.

"People didn't know what they were looking for in a woman bodybuilder," she recalled. "I thought, to set a new trend, I'd come in defined. I didn't have that much muscle, but what I had was defined. At that contest, they went for the muscle mass. I got bad reviews but it set a trend. Now girls are coming in leaner, more defined."

It's hard to believe that the woman who stepped out on the Las Vegas Caesars Palace stage to win the America (lightweight) less than two years and almost 20 muscular pounds later was once underdeveloped. And those arms—you've seen those massive muscle bellies, bellies full of curling strength! So I asked (nonchalantly), "How'd you build those arms in such a short time, Mary?"

"I don't want to get into details," she replied.

After the disappointing second place in the Robby Robinson event, it was almost a year

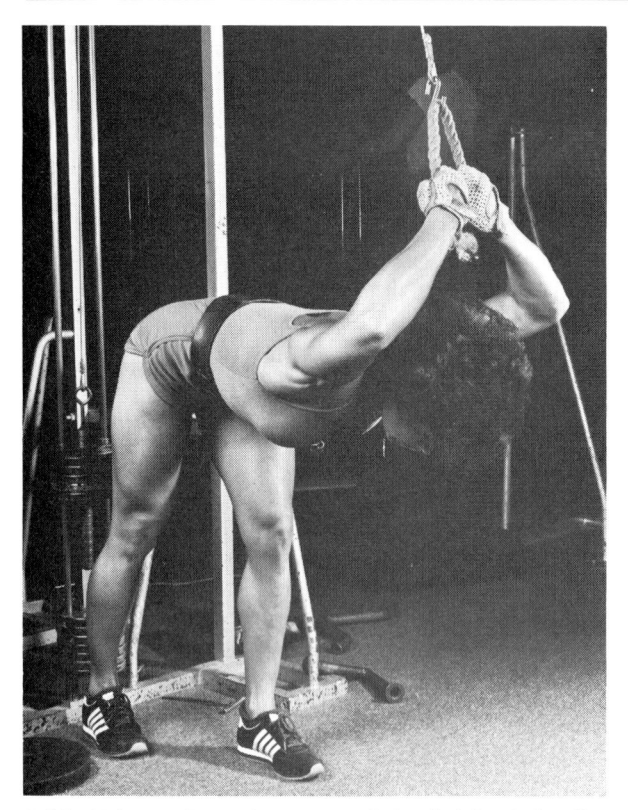

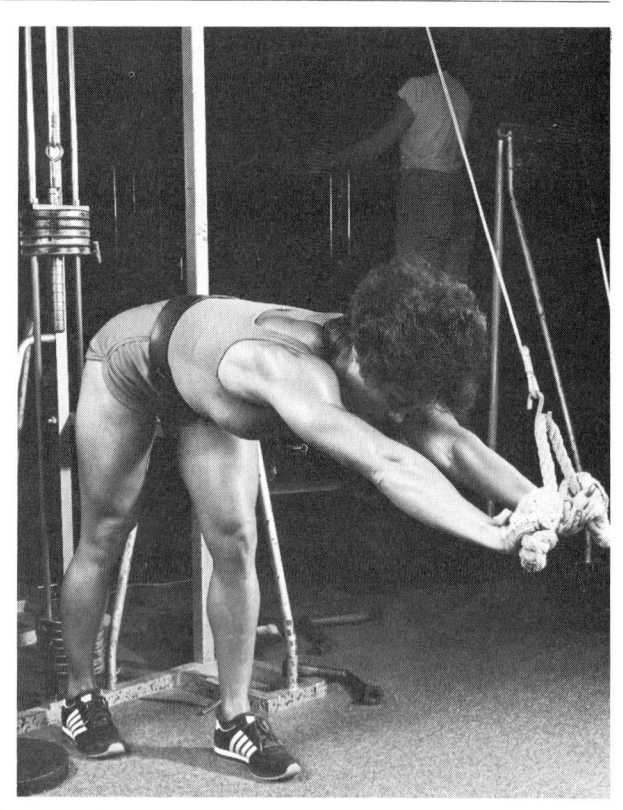

Cable Triceps Extension—start, left; finish, right. "For the long head of the triceps, you can do extensions as illustrated here. Be sure to bend your arms more at the start, however."

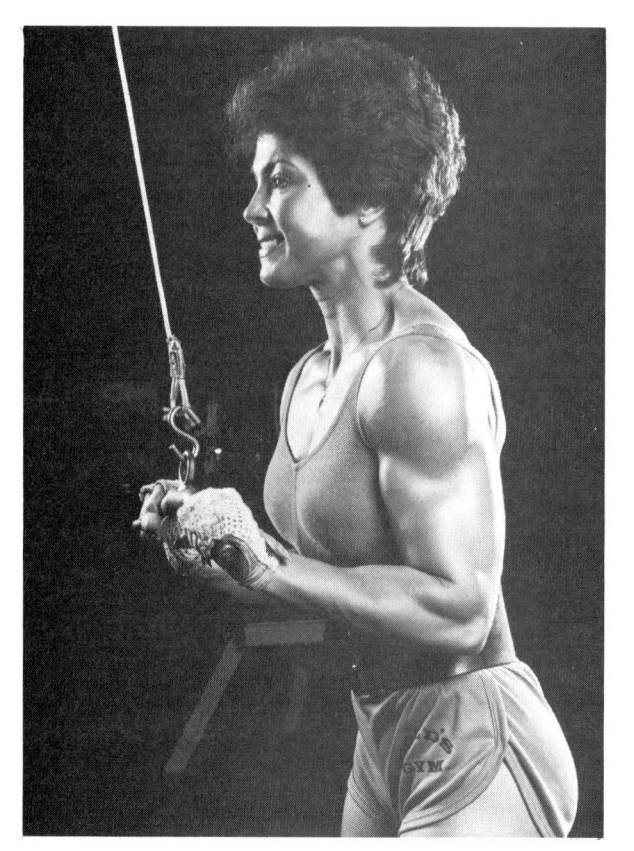

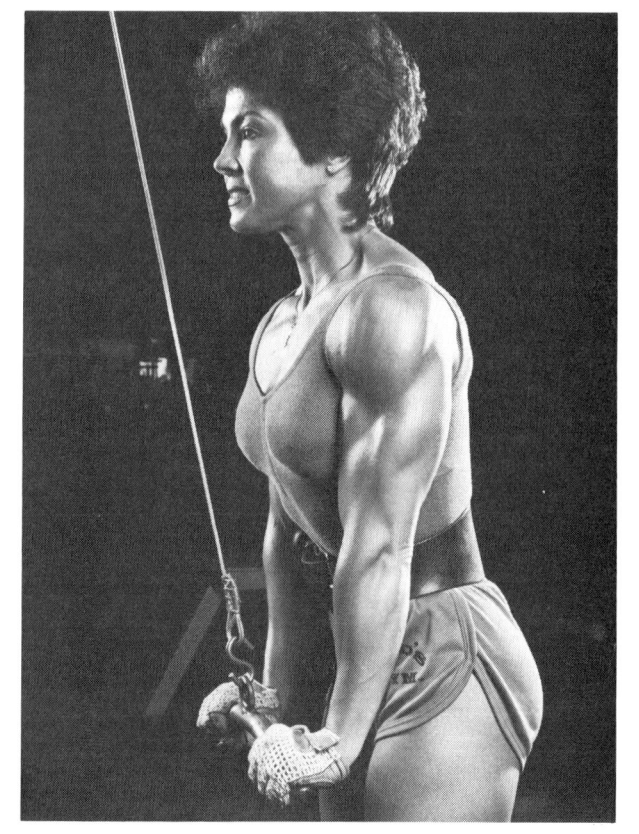

Triceps Pressdown—start, left; finish, right. "Lean slightly forward and keep your elbows tightly against your sides as you do a full pressdown—from your chin to your thighs."

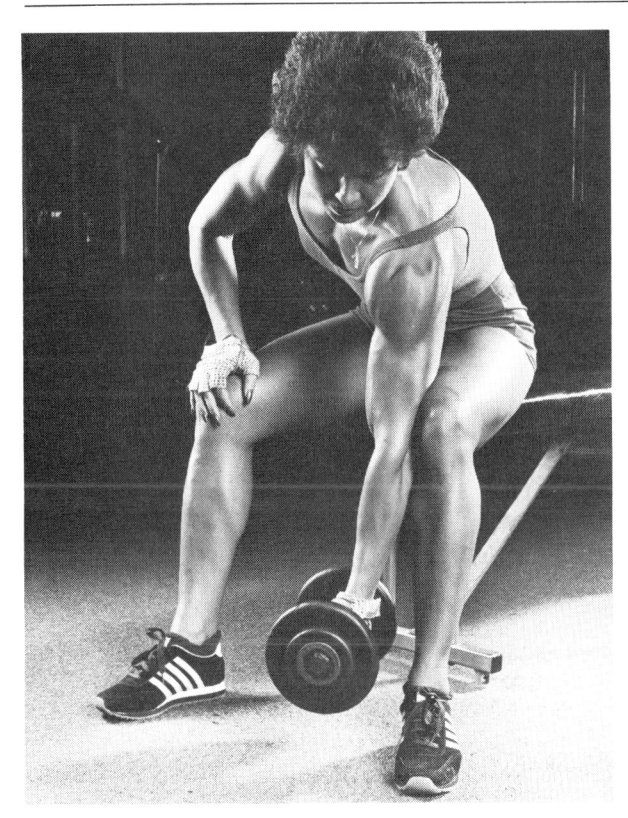

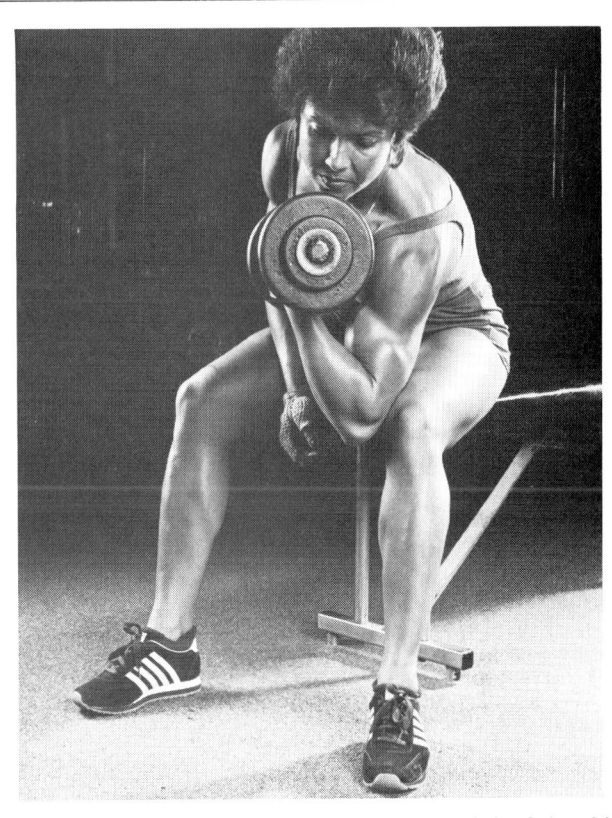

Concentration Curl—start, left; finish, right. "Brace the working arm against the inside of your knee and think 'peak' as you slowly curl the dumbbell completely up."

before Mary competed again. Her hiatus was no vacation. It was a time-out because of a back injury. "After I had the back surgery, I went into a deep depression because I remembered what I could do in the gym before, and after the surgery I couldn't even lift my leg. I laid off for seven months to get rehabilitated. The muscles in my left leg had begun to atrophy. My reflexes were gone in my left foot because my sciatic nerve was pinched for so long."

Her next contest was the 1981 Ms. Western America. Mary was ready and heavy (108 pounds). She had what the judges wanted—more size. "I knew I had to gain a little size, to build the density. That contest was just a prep for the America. I hadn't been onstage for a year. I wanted to get the feel of the stage, get a feel for the audience so I could capture them. I'm not really interested in who I'm competing against. I'm there to demonstrate what I've done with my physique, so I'm fearful of no one."

"Especially with those arms," I said, seizing the opportunity. She laughed. I was getting to her. Or maybe it was the half cup of red wine vinegar she had doused her salad with. She was loosening up.

"Look, I know you can't tell me all your secrets. Just tell me what you can," I said with a smile. I hoped it didn't seem like groveling. She leaned forward as if we were two spies on a confidential mission somewhere in the Middle East. Then she started talking.

"I have certain tricks which involve working the tie-in muscles that make my physique look prettier. There are certain angles that I do on the cables that make the muscle longer, rather than building those short, squatty-looking muscles. I work through a full range of motion plus some. Like on Cable Triceps Extensions. At the end of the pull, I turn out the palms of my hand. This isolates and contracts the triceps more than doing the Extensions alone. I can tell you some things, but I can't tell you everything."

Once started, Mary rolled with the momentum. "A lot of attributes can't be developed through exercises. They're just heredity, like splits in the biceps. People are mistaken when they say anyone can get split biceps with a certain exercise. Look at Sergio Oliva—he has big arms but he doesn't have split biceps. He's impressive anyway. I'm more into symmetry. Some people don't think you can have both muscularity and symmetry, but I disagree. To solve symmetry problems at times requires putting mass on your body—not necessarily stripping excess mass but putting

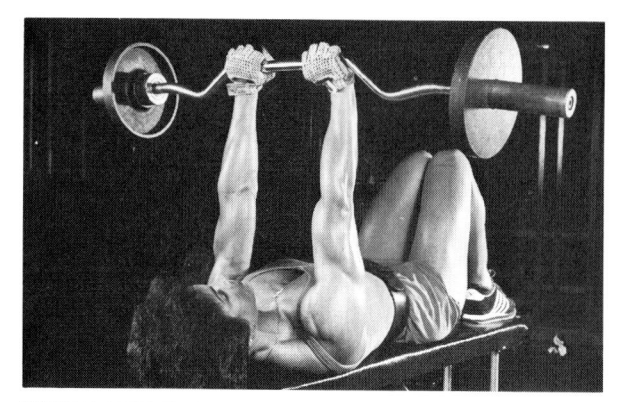

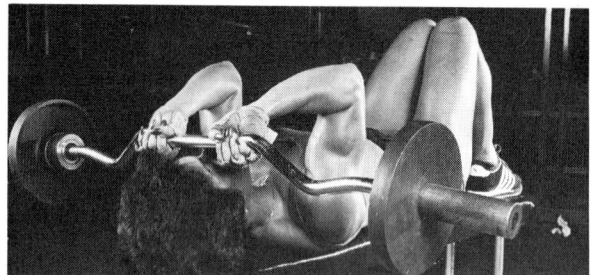

Lying Triceps Extension—start, top; finish, bottom. "The secret to this movement is to move the elbows as little as possible, which places maximum stress on the triceps."

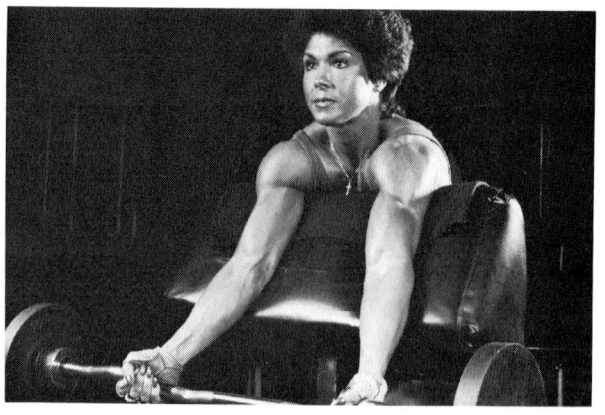

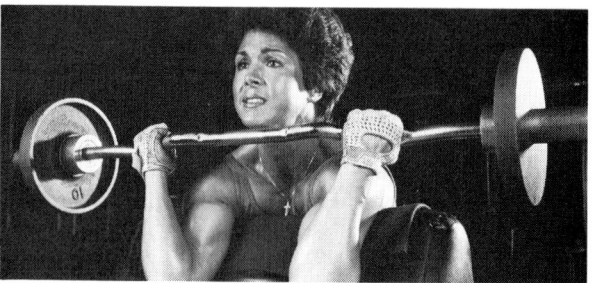

Preacher Curl—start, top; finish, bottom. "Be sure to get a full extension at the bottom and then curl the bar slowly up to a point right under your chin."

mass on where it belongs. And to build size, you've got to work heavy."

To Mary Roberts, working heavy means more than just lifting heavy poundage, although she does that, too. Heavy training means working a split routine six days a week. Two and a half hours in the morning and the same length of time at night. The first three days of the week she uses heavy weights. The last three days the weights are much lighter. "When I feel strong I can do Alternate Dumbbell Curls with 40-pound dumbbells. If I'm dieting, I'm lucky if I can do 20 pounds. It all depends on how I feel.

"Sometimes I go to the gym, start to train and I don't feel like training, so I don't train. My body is telling me something. It's telling me I need a rest," Mary explained. Sound familiar? It ought to—that's the Weider Instinctive Training Principle. It means listening to your body. For many people, it also means avoiding overtraining, preventing injuries, and getting the most out of your workout when you're feeling up.

The Weider Instinctive Training Principle plays a major role in Mary's arm training. For example, to train her arms (biceps and triceps), she does 15–18 sets (6–8 repetitions per set) on heavy days and 10 sets on light days. For biceps, the total number of sets is made up of some combination of Concentration Curls, Preacher Curls with an EZ-curl bar, Cable Curls, Curls with an Olympic bar (done while standing) and Alternating Dumbbell Curls. Exactly how many sets of each exercise is determined by how Mary feels on that particular day. And the weights she'll choose to lift, again, depend on her strength level at the time.

Another interesting thing Mary revealed was that she trains her forearms four days a week. She recognizes that arm size is made up of balanced biceps and triceps development, and also that upper arm size must balance with forearm size.

There are some things Mary keeps secret, like the personal training tricks all experienced bodybuilders have, and there are other things she considers unimportant. When asked how big her arms were, her reply was quick and firm. "I do not measure my body at all. I just look in the mirror. I don't get into measurements."

I don't know how big they are either because I didn't accost Mary with a measuring tape, but they're sure a lot bigger than nine inches. Whatever they measure is irrelevant, because it's obvious that her training techniques work. Her formula for full, muscular arms is simple: high-powered workouts tempered by the Weider Instinctive Training Principle. With Weider and weights, success can also be yours! □

Energize Your Legs!

by Rachel McLish

No doubt about it! From the sweeping curve of the biceps femoris to the dramatic tautness of the sartorius; from the deeply etched grooves of the vastus lateralis and medialis to the crystal cut of the gastrocnemius, there is *nothing* more impressive to behold—and to have—than a pair of beautifully muscled, shapely legs.

For as long as I can remember, I have been fascinated by well-developed legs. Even as a child, the first thing that I noticed about top ballet artists, gymnasts and dancers was their strong, powerful legs. Great legs still hold their magic appeal and remain a priority in my training.

Maybe you've always wanted super legs, too, but thought it was an unreachable goal. Well, it isn't. You *can* develop legs that you can be really proud of, but it takes strenuous, carefully planned workouts.

You have to get involved. In order to put your all into a workout, there has to be some kind of goal. My leg workouts have become easier, more enjoyable and a whole lot more rewarding because I *visualize* the end result of my labors. I concentrate on the outcome: strong, shapely, show-stopping legs! Focusing on the desired effect puts a great deal of meaning into every grueling set and each drop of perspiration, because I know that they're bringing me that much closer to leg perfection! And despite my sweat-soaked workout clothes, that makes me feel absolutely *beautiful!* By adopting my leg routine—along with this visualization technique—you'll experience shapely gains like never before!

I've found, through trial and error, that standard exercise techniques aren't really the most effective. Achieving the ultimate in results often requires some alterations in form. An odd angle here, a different foot position there, and suddenly you've made a dramatic change in the effectiveness of a movement. When it comes to bodybuilding, little things do mean a lot.

So when you try out my leg workout, which I've outlined below, pay close attention to the form that I use in each exercise. It's different for a reason. And if a well-meaning—but annoying, just the same—exercise instructor descends upon you and says, "You're doing that all wrong," tell him or her that this is how Rachel McLish told you to do it. Then keep on building those legs!

Lunges—I begin my leg workout by warming up with a few Lunges, done in the conventional manner while holding a very light weight. Then I do a series of Lunges using my own technique. I visually pick a spot on the floor in front of me and reach for it with my lead-off leg, so that I feel a good stretch in both legs. As I perform the movement, I simultaneously contract the buttocks muscle of the back leg and the quadriceps muscles of the front leg, keeping the back leg straight. I then return to the starting position and repeat the action, leading with the other leg. The continuous shift in bodyweight will add resistance, so you only need to use a light weight.

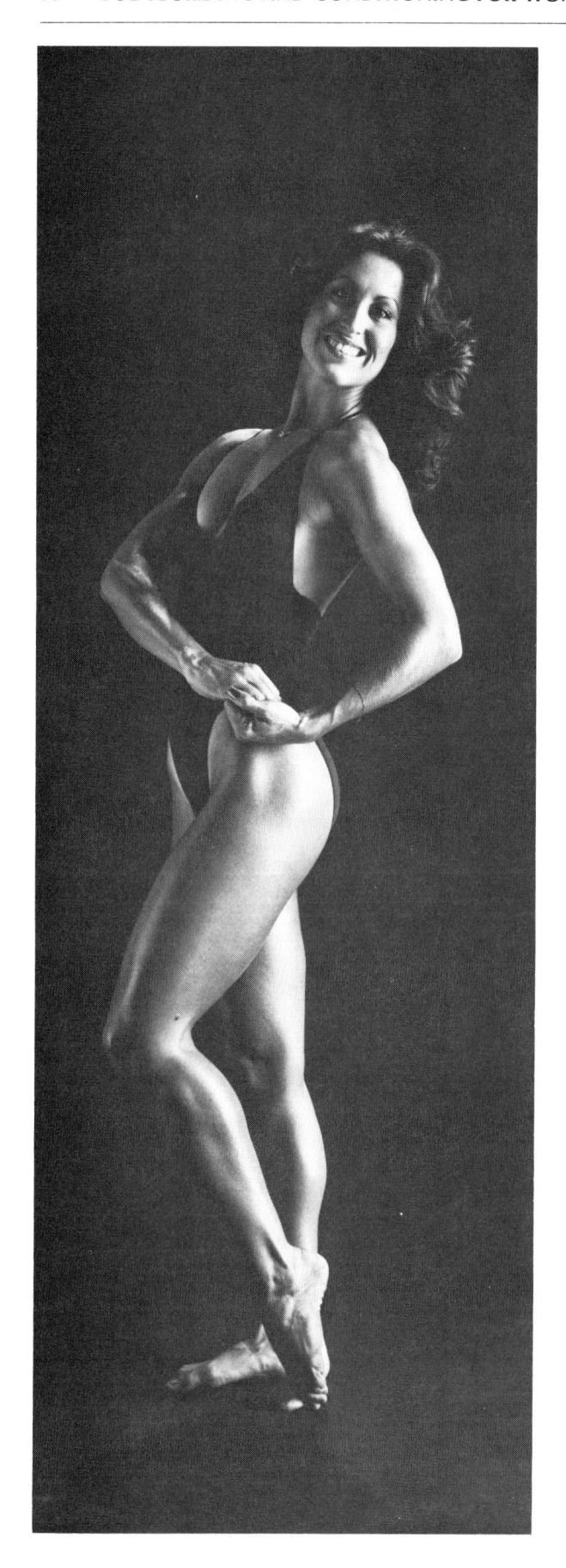

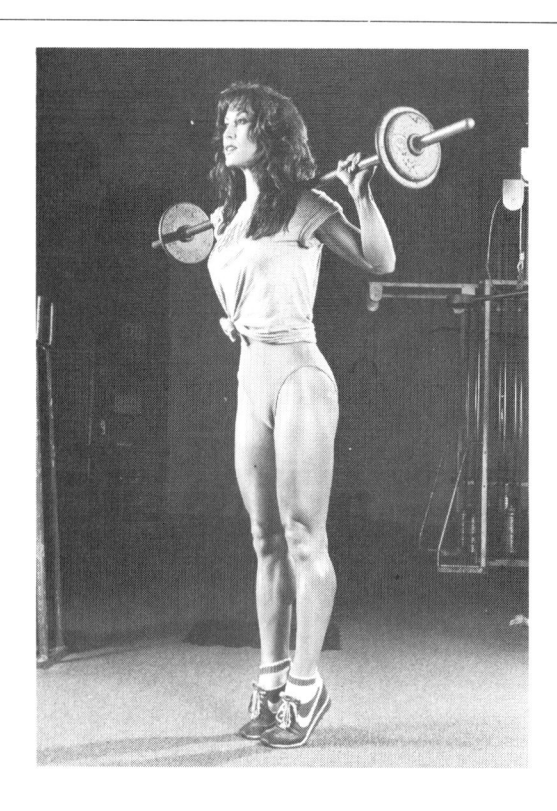

Squats and Leg Press—These exercises, along with Hack Squats, build power as well as mass. I prefer the Leg Press because I can use heavier weight, the injury factor is almost completely eliminated, and I can stimulate different areas by varying my foot position. With feet pointing out, I experience a gratifying contraction in the vastus lateralis up to the inner glutes. Stimulation of the inner thigh and outer glutes is achieved by pointing the feet inward. These variations are effective, but you should take it even further by bringing your own creativity into your leg training.

Leg Curls—Your old friend, the leg curl machine, provides great exercise for the hamstrings—with the added bonus of firming and rounding the buttocks. But even vicious sets with heavy weights will have no merit if you don't concentrate on contraction and form. Remember to keep your hips as close to the bench as possible. Your hips will inevitably come up a little when you raise the weight, but try your utmost to control them when you lower the weight. I get a superior contraction this way.

ENERGIZE YOUR LEGS! 97

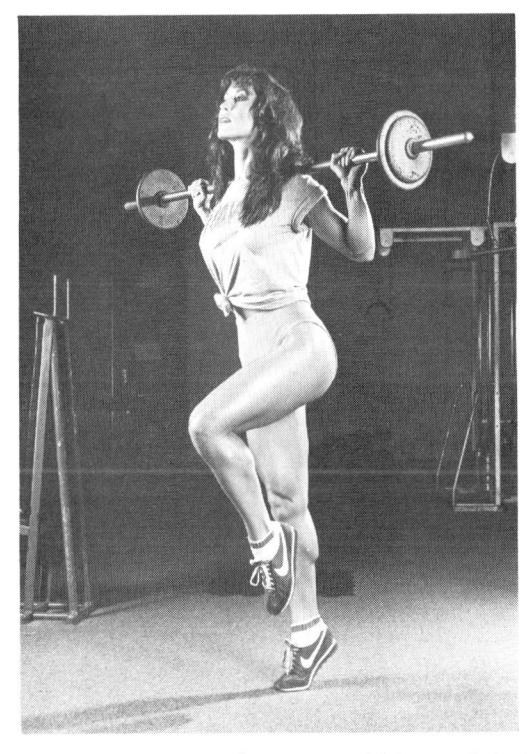

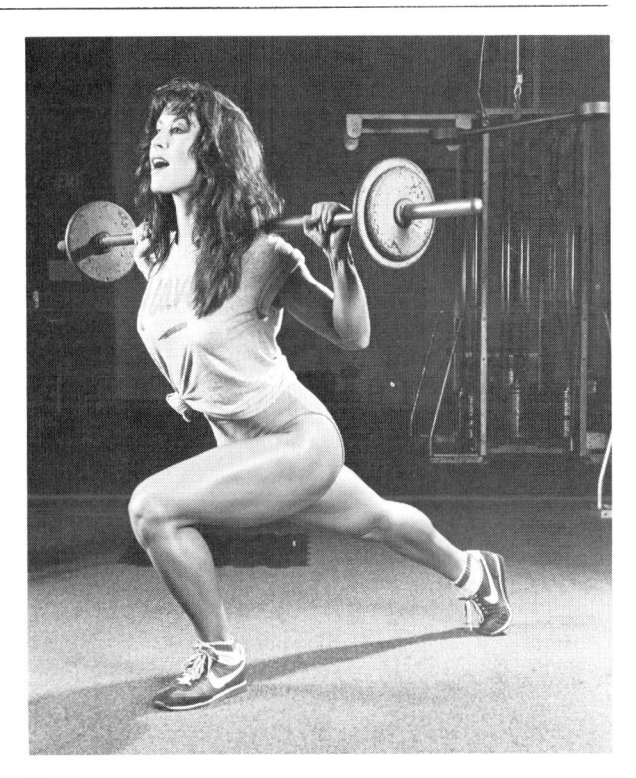

Lunge—start, opposite page; mid-lunge, left; finish, right.

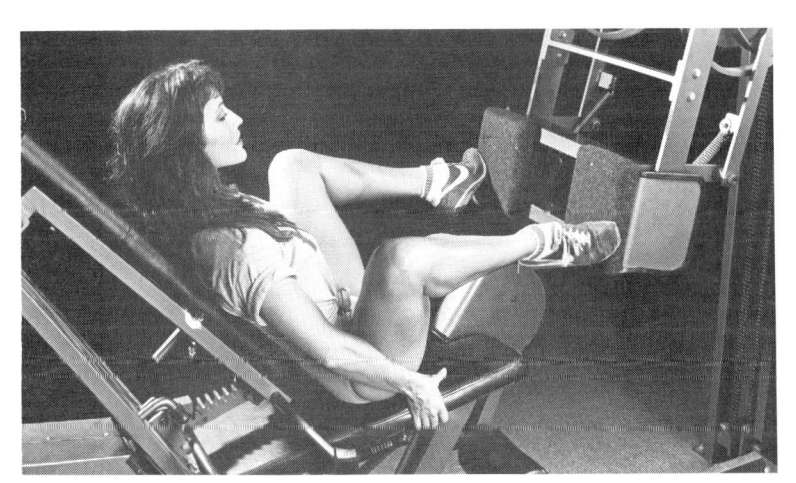

Leg Press—start, above; finish, right. Note that you can vary foot positions for excellent effects.

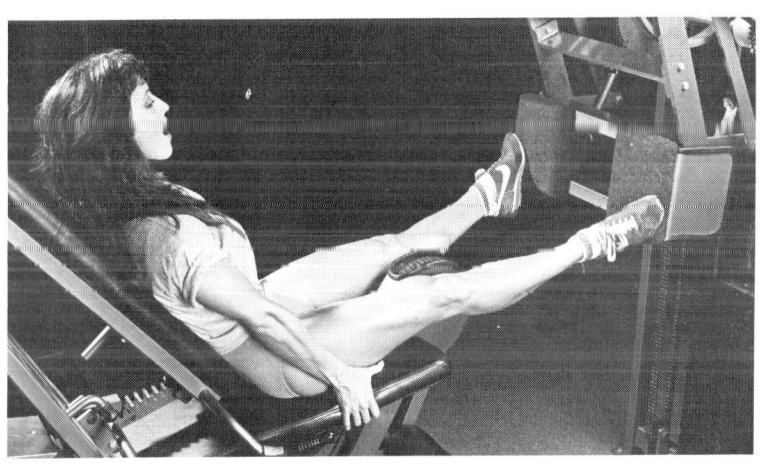

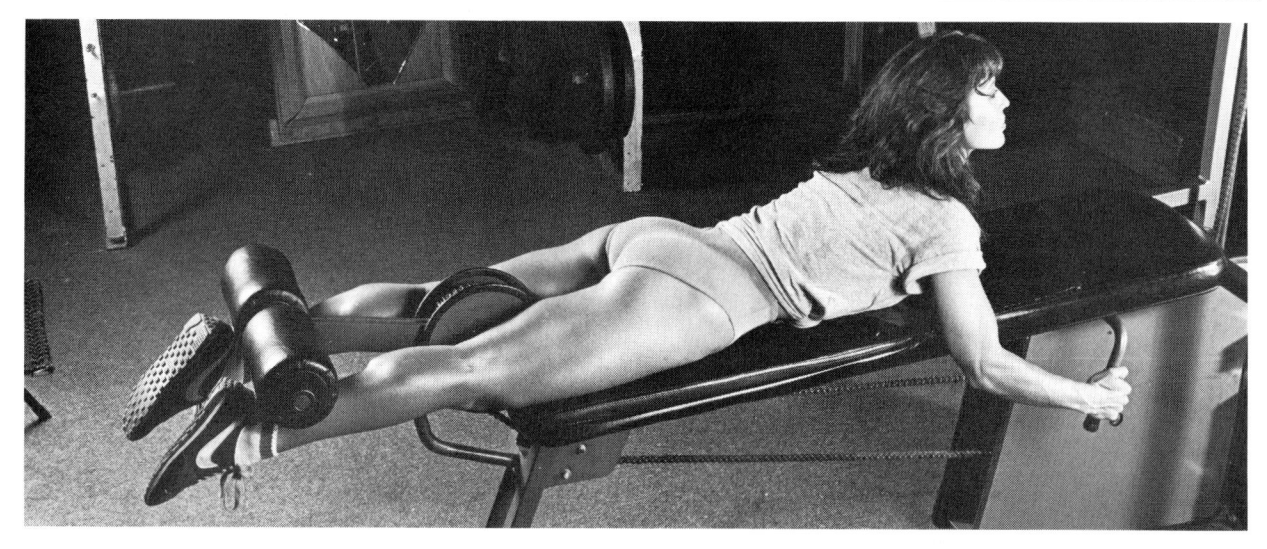

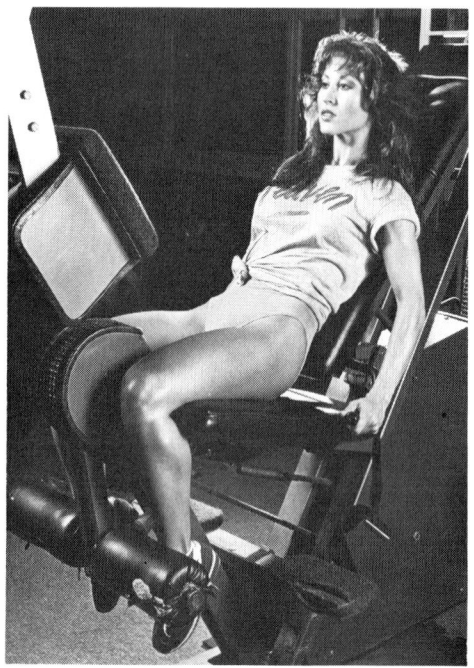

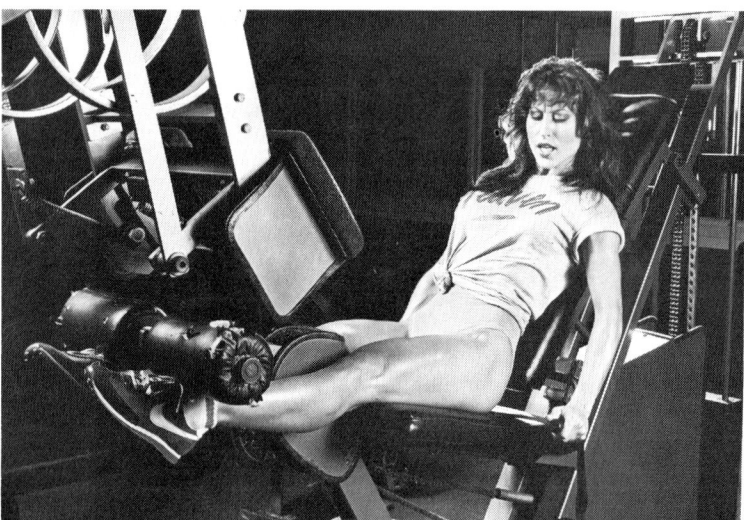

Top, start for Leg Curls. Leg Extension—start, left; finish, right.

Experimenting on this machine, I've discovered another way to isolate the leg biceps: upon completion of the positive, upward movement, hold the contraction for a couple of seconds, and then contract the buttock of one leg in an effort to bring that leg past the initial end point. Then lower the weight and repeat with the other leg.

Leg Extensions—It's almost impossible not to get a good contraction on an adequate leg extension machine. But, again, you can benefit from variety. Raise the weight with both legs and lower it with one. Concentrate on completely flexing the frontal thigh muscles. Invaluable to superior leg development, Leg Extensions are a fantastic way to get that last bit of effort out of your leg muscles.

This routine isn't primarily designed to bulk up your legs, but rather to polish their appearance. Keep the reps high (up to 15) and do three sets of each exercise in circuit style. Use light to moderate weights, but not so light that the exercises feel too easy. By concentrating on the contractions, you'll make light-weight workouts as effective and intense as heavy workouts! I hope my routine stimulates your interest in leg training. It's vital for total fitness and beauty—and for "flex appeal."

These Legs Stop Traffic

by Bill Dobbins

Saturday night, Florida—On a taut canvas, not really of official dimensions, two men square off. It's a "Bad Man" competition, allowing stevedores, truck drivers, fishermen, cowboys and other would-be tough guys the chance to square off in the ring. Titles here are irrelevant . . . there's a more primal motivation fueling this enterprise, and nothing short of a miracle can stop the combatants or cheering sections.

Then Georgia Miller Fudge and husband Dick enter. In a few short minutes the crowd stops paying attention to the battle in the ring. Instead, a crowd rapidly forms around Georgia. Flashbulbs pop, autographs are sought. Some tough guys merely stare.

"It was incredible," Dick Fudge recalls. "But everywhere Georgia goes, people recognize her. In whatever part of the country, it doesn't matter whether Georgia visits a shopping mall, or goes to the movies, people stop and stare, whisper, point at her.

"That night in Florida, she almost caused a riot. As soon as we walked in the door, people started coming up to her—'Hi, Georgia.' 'How're you doing, Georgia?' One guy started taking pictures, and soon everybody was standing on their seats to see her, ignoring the fight. One Hell's Angel came over and said, 'Hey flex those arms. They really turn me on.'"

However, no matter how much attention Georgia's arm development attracts, Dick agrees that her legs are what really stop traffic.

"I remember once walking behind Georgia and Kay Baxter just to see how people reacted to them. They were both in short-shorts and I was afraid they were going to cause a traffic accident. I also remember the first time I saw Georgia— she was wearing a halter top and shorts and I practically flew across the room to meet her. Even then, her legs were fantastic."

Georgia takes pride in her long, shapely legs; however, as a bodybuilder she is aware that the same qualities that make her legs attractive to the general public also make it difficult for her to develop the ideal proportions necessary to win top-level competitions.

"Having long legs makes it hard to build enough mass," explains Georgia. "It's exactly the same problem tall male bodybuilders face. A tall man can be massive and still not have well-proportioned thighs. I guess that's why there are so few outstanding bodybuilders over six feet tall. For a woman, the cut-off point seems to be around 5'7". If a woman bodybuilder is taller than that, she'll find it difficult to appear proportioned."

Of course, once a tall bodybuilder develops the right size, the added length of line tends to provide outstanding symmetry. So Georgia feels it's just a matter of time and training until she

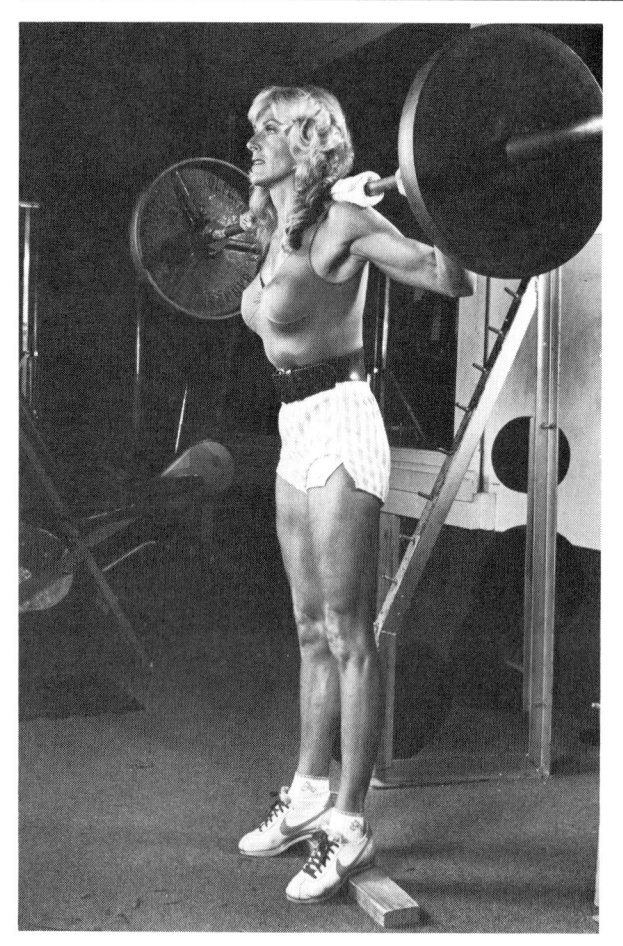

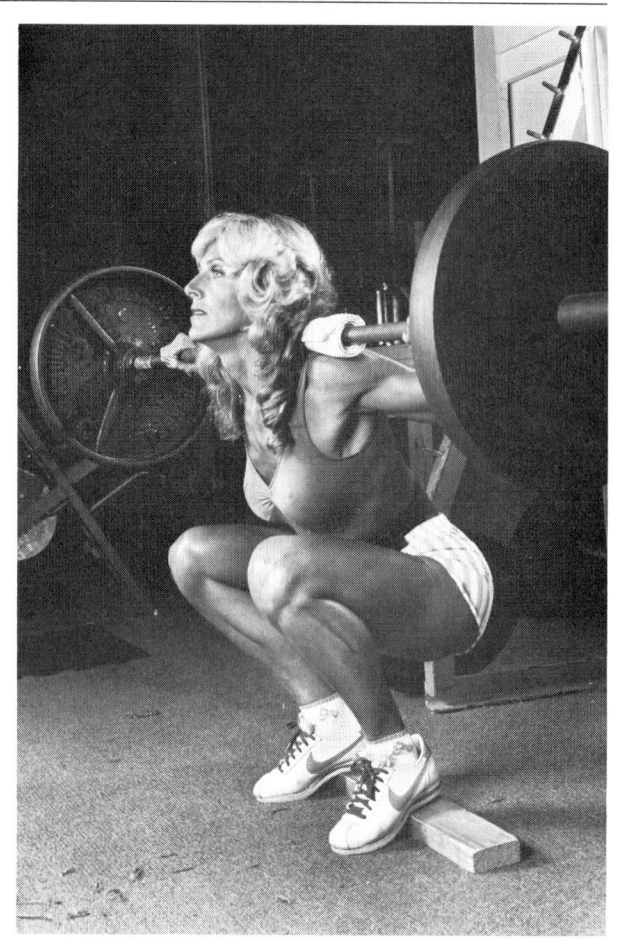

Squat—start, left; finish, right. Keep back straight and elevate heels to keep stress on front thighs.

acquires those extra inches that will make her a consistent winner of international competitions.

"One problem I've noticed," Georgia adds, "is that I tend to lose size in my thighs while on a contest diet. This isn't just fat loss, but a loss in muscle tissue. I have to experiment by dieting different ways, or maybe by adding more aerobic exercise, so that I can get cut up without any loss of lean body mass."

Another new approach Georgia uses to build her legs involves the concept—attributed to Vince Gironda—that "bodybuilding is illusion." In this philosophy it doesn't matter how large or small any given bodypart actually is as long as it *looks* right.

"I've made more progress recently by concentrating on building the lower part of my thighs, down near the knee," Georgia says. "Too much taper makes the thigh look smaller than it is. So I've changed my leg routine to better develop the rectus femoris and the vastus medialis."

Georgia's leg training has been somewhat handicapped because a knee injury suffered in high school prevents her from doing very heavy Squats.

"Anyway," Dick says, "my belief is that women tend to exaggerate the amount of weight they use for Squats. I hear and read about women using 250 to 275 pounds. But if these women were doing what I considered a good full Squat—not all the way down, but well below parallel—this amount of weight would drive them right down to the floor."

Dick has always taught Georgia that she should do Squats strictly and correctly to achieve total thigh development, rather than attempt to break world powerlifting records. Many women, along with their male counterparts, often forget that training like powerlifters, if carried beyond a certain point, makes them look like powerlifters, which won't help them win bodybuilding contests.

"I've done Squats from Day One," explains Georgia, "and they have helped me immensely. But now I've replaced some sets of Squats with

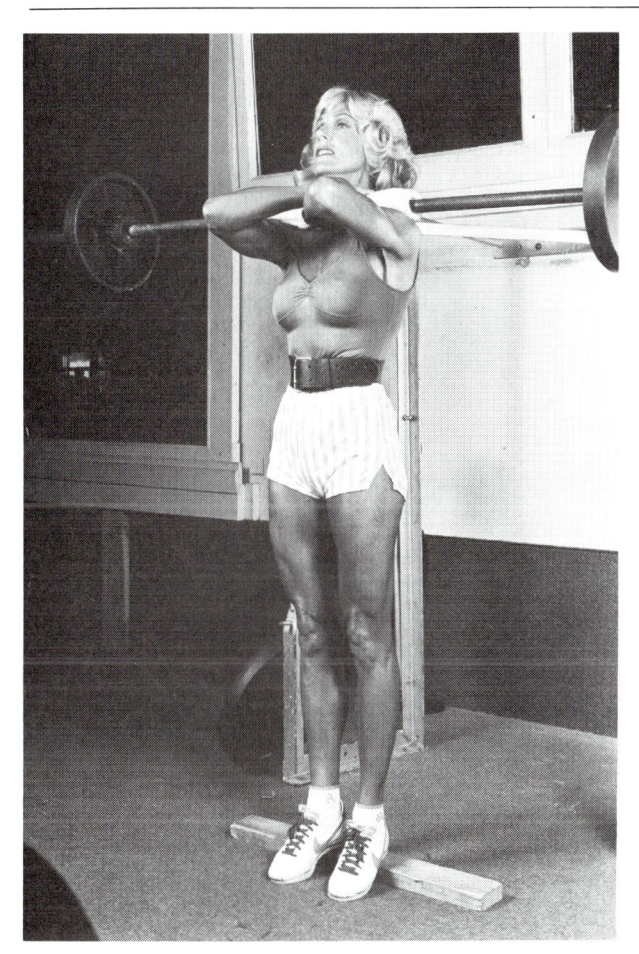

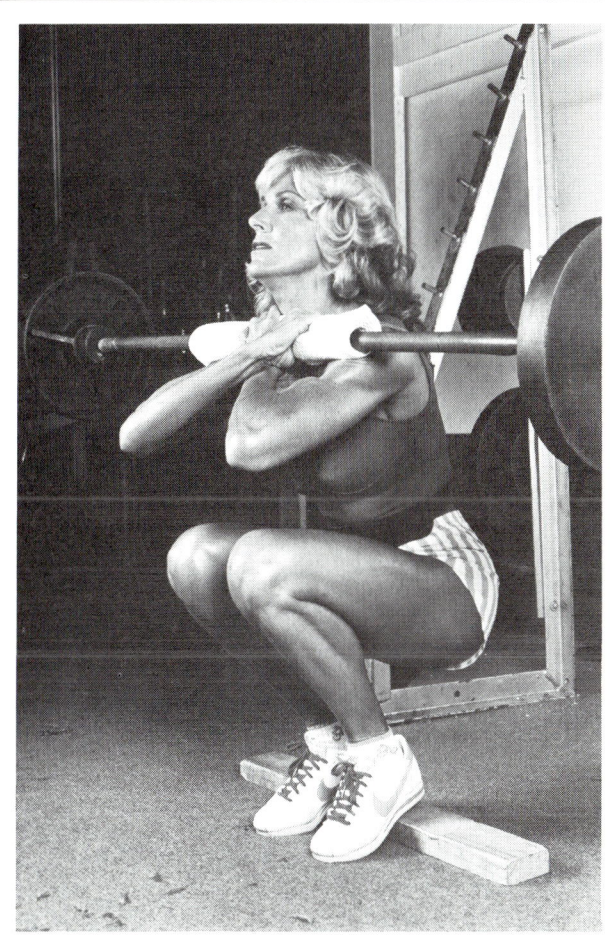

Front Squat—start, left; finish, right. This is how it is meant to be done.

several sets of Front Squats. I feel that these allow me to better develop the lower thighs."

After only a few months on this routine, Georgia and Dick already see results; however, they have also found that when one thing changes for the better, another can change for the worse.

"When I did a lot of Hack Squats," Georgia says, "I had a very good split in the front of my quadriceps. Since I have been doing Front Squats instead, my lower quadriceps are bigger, but the split is less well-defined. There are so many variables involved in bodybuilding, it's hard to say which one causes a change. This is why it takes so many years to figure out what works for each individual. No wonder older male bodybuilders like Frank Zane, Chris Dickerson and Albert Beckles do so well—they've had 15 or 20 years of training experience to help them understand all the variables. None of the women in bodybuilding has anywhere near that much experience."

One exercise Georgia doesn't do is the Leg Press. Although many bodybuilders feel that this leg exercise is a *primary* mass builder, Dick Fudge's personal opinion is that Leg Presses contribute very little to the right kind of bodybuilding development.

"I have two vertical Leg Press machines in my gym," he says, "and I've been watching bodybuilders do Leg Presses for 30 years. I think this is an exercise you can do forever and still have nothing to show. It's good for glutes and upper thighs, but that doesn't develop a very aesthetic leg. Georgia tried them for a while, but they didn't do anything for her."

The one problem Georgia has experienced with Front Squats comes from the fact that women have less front deltoid development than men. As a result, women often have trouble finding a "shelf" on which to comfortably and securely rest the bar. Carla Dunlap has also noted this problem. This means that women often must use less weight than they'd like to, but this makes them concentrate even more fully on correct technique.

102 BODYBUILDING AND CONDITIONING FOR WOMEN

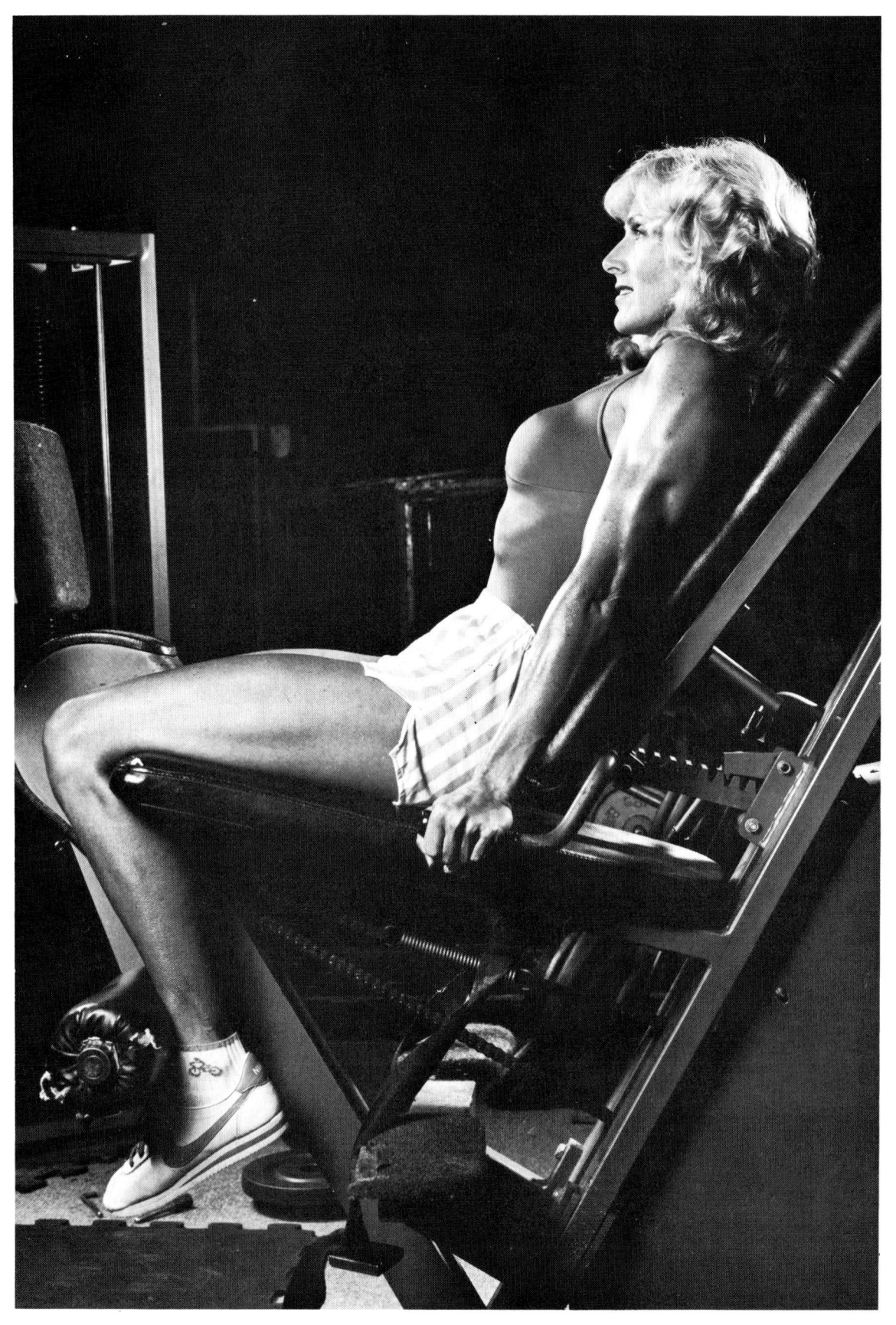

Thigh Extensions help shape and define the quadriceps muscles.

"Although Front Squats present some difficulties," Georgia says adamantly, "they have worked so well for me that it's worth the extra effort."

Actually, Georgia uses relatively few exercises in her leg routine. In recent months, these were: Squats, Front Squats, Leg Extensions, Lunges and Leg Curls. However, she uses two arrangements of these exercises to produce different results. Until recently, her leg workout looked like this:

1. Squats (three or four sets, seven reps)
2. Front Squats (six supersets)
3. Leg Extensions (six supersets)
4. Lunges (six sets)
5. Leg Curls (six sets)

"This arrangement was great for thigh definition because the Front Squats and Leg Extensions produced continuous stress on my quadriceps," Georgia says. "However, we decided that if I want more size on my lower

Lunge—start, left; finish, below. Compare Georgia's technique, which attempts to lengthen stride as much as possible, with Rachel's Lunge on pages 96–97.

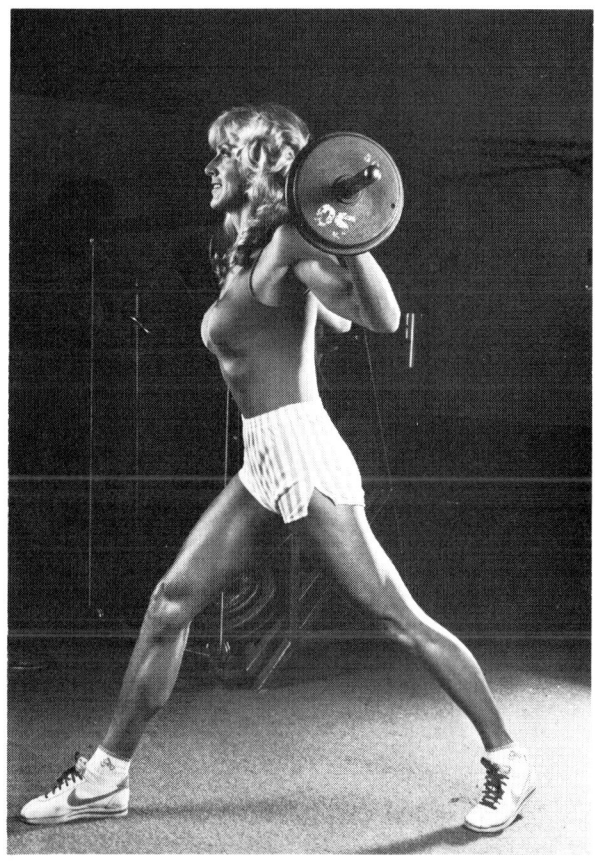

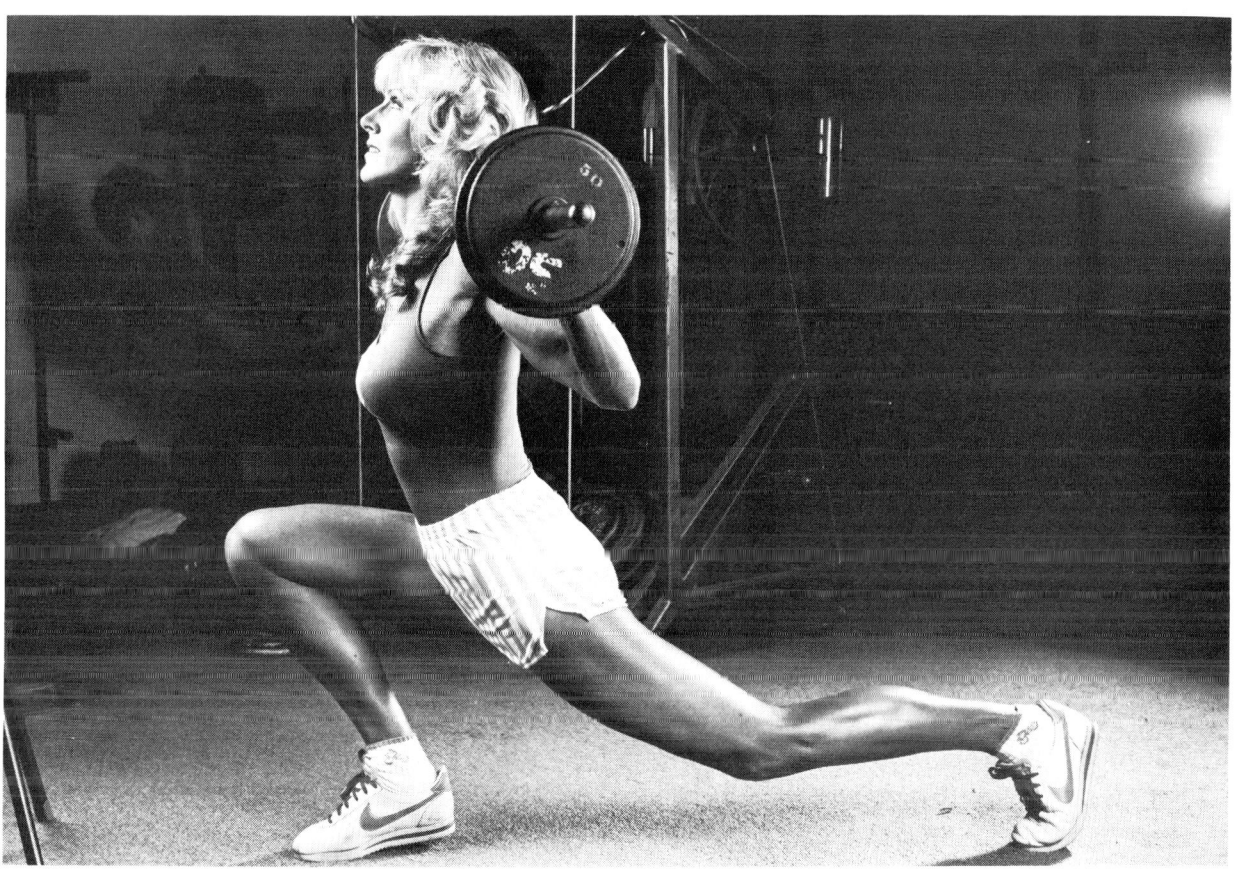

thighs, it would be better to separate these two movements."

Currently, Georgia's arrangement of leg exercises is as follows:

1. Squats (three or four sets, seven reps)
2. Front Squats (six supersets)
3. Lunges (six supersets)
4. Leg Extensions (six sets)
5. Leg Curls (six sets)

"I built an Incline Leg Extension machine for Georgia," Dick explains, "that lets her work her quadriceps through a full range of motion and achieve full contraction without locking out and holding at the top. This means she can work very hard without risking strain on her knee."

When Georgia does Lunges, she takes as long a stride as possible. Using a 90-pound barbell, she works one leg at a time, finishing her reps with that leg before shifting to the other.

"I try to feel the Lunges in the back of the leg and the glutes. At the first Miss Olympia contest, George Snyder told me that my one major weakness was lack of hardness in this area."

"I don't think Georgia has any major weaknesses any more," says Dick Fudge, "although I think she can get better. One training advantage Georgia has is that her body responds quickly to different routines. If we change her routine we see a difference in her physique within a few weeks. So we can figure out pretty quickly what works and what doesn't."

Another advantage Georgia boasts is having Dick as her coach. Bodybuilding is one of the few sports in which competitors do not get regular coaching. Gymnasts, football players, swimmers and other athletes all benefit from coaches, who constantly monitor form and correct technique.

"Dick watches me train, makes sure I work hard enough, judges the results and helps me change my routine," Georgia says. "He's been in bodybuilding so long that he's seen everybody and everything, and he always has a good perception of what will work for me. I can't imagine where I'd be now without his help."

"I still think it would be good if Georgia trained with somebody else for a while," Dick claims. "When we train together, we experience the typical husband-and-wife problem: She has a tendency to argue with me when I make suggestions. If she were training with a woman who works out really hard, I feel Georgia would train with more intensity, and move farther into the 'Pain Zone,' as Joe Weider calls it."

"It's true," says Georgia, "I'm so competitive that just *seeing* a woman bodybuilder who trains hard makes me want to go into the gym and train even harder. So Dick is probably right—but I wouldn't want to train solely with someone else and not have the benefit of my husband's coaching."

Besides, in addition to being Georgia's husband and coach, Dick Fudge is also her greatest fan. From the moment he first saw her, he believed she had the potential to be the best woman bodybuilder in the world.

"Georgia," Dick says, "has legs that, in terms of symmetry and shape, are the female equivalent of Steve Reeves' or Dick Haislop's. Year by year, she is adding the mass that will eventually give her ideal proportions as well. When that happens, I don't think there is a woman in the world who could beat her."□